A Guide for Beginning Psychotherapists

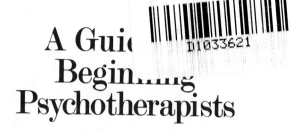

JOAN S. ZARO

*Associate Administrative Officer,
Professional Affairs, American
Psychological Association,
Washington, D.C.*

ROLAND BARACH

*Research Associate, Department
of Psychology, University of
Washington, Seattle, and Staff
Associate, Biofeedback and
Stress Management Institute,
Seattle*

DEBORAH JO NEDELMAN

*Staff Associate, Pacific
Psychological Services, Seattle*

IRWIN S. DREIBLATT

*Co-director, Pacific
Psychological Services, Seattle,
and Affiliate Associate Professor
of Psychology and Clinical
Associate Professor of Psychiatry
and Behavioral Sciences,
University of Washington,
Seattle*

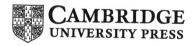

CAMBRIDGE
UNIVERSITY PRESS

PUBLISHED BY PRESS SYNDICATE OF THE UNIVERSITY OF CAMBRIDGE
The Pitt Building, Trumpington Street, Cambridge CB2 1RP, United Kingdom

CAMBRIDGE UNIVERSITY PRESS
The Edinburgh Building, Cambridge CB2 2RU, United Kingdom
40 West 20th Street, New York, NY 10011-4211, USA
10 Stamford Road, Oakleigh, Melbourne 3166, Australia

First published 1977
Reprinted 1978, 1979 (twice), 1980, 1982, 1983 (twice), 1985,
1987 (twice), 1988, 1990, 1991, 1993 (twice), 1994, 1995,
1996, 1997

Printed in the United States of America

Typeset in Primer

A catalogue record for this book is available from the British Library

Library of Congress Cataloguing-in-Publication Data is available

ISBN 0-521-29230-1 paperback

Contents

Contents

Contents

Preface

This book provides a broad introduction to the practical complexities of learning psychotherapeutic skills. It was written in response to the needs of beginning therapists for reassurance and concrete guidance, and in response to the need of the authors for a reference text in their roles as practicum supervisors. In our experiences with neophyte therapists we repeatedly encountered their feelings of impatience, self-doubt, frustration, and disappointment. The demands for performance on beginners are great; such demands come both from within students themselves and from the training setting.

Although it is not possible, and probably not desirable, to escape these painful experiences entirely, we hope this book will help ease the individual's transition from student to professional therapist. We have discussed many of the practical problems that are commonly encountered during the introduction to interviewing, treatment assessment, and psychotherapy. Some of the student's upsetting and possibly harmful mistakes may be avoided through exposure to these typical problem areas, and through reading our discussions and suggestions.

We have tried to carry out this task in a practical, concrete manner, with a student-oriented rather than client-oriented approach. We have raised problematic issues, offered suggestions about what to do and how to do it, and relied on a liberal use of examples that the students may use as models in problem solving. Admittedly, these questions are complex and the answers cannot be simple. This book represents no substitute for supervised experience in the development of a solid individual sense of competence as a psychotherapist. Moreover, this is not an attempt to provide the thorough knowledge base in normal and abnormal behavior, assessment, and treatment that is essential to the student's preparation as a clinician.

Clinical training ideally involves sensitive and timely discussions of the issues raised in this book. However, the immediate demands on both student and supervisor while providing treatment in a training setting often override the need for attention to personal concerns and broad practical guidance. Thus the authors intend this book to be used by supervisors as an adjunct to the supervision sessions, and as a basis for more in-depth role playing and class discussion.

The basic tools discussed in this book are intended to be useful to students and supervisors in a variety of disciplines and work settings. We believe that the practical psychotherapeutic skills, and the practicalities of learning them, are common across professional and theoretical boundaries, including clinical and counseling psychology, social work, psychiatry, pastoral counseling, psychiatric nursing, and educational and school psychology. Although most students at the graduate level are exposed to the knowledge and theory of their fields, this may do little to prepare them for practicum training. Here they all face the experience of attempting to apply this new knowledge to actual clinical problems.

We take seriously the great personal and professional changes involved in learning to become a therapist and hope that this book in some way facilitates the often painful, always awkward experience – for the student, the supervisor, and the client.

We acknowledge our debt to the students we have supervised, and to their willingness to share with us the anxieties, the self-doubts, and the variety of other feelings they experienced during their struggling first attempts at therapy. We are also certainly indebted to the clients served by these students. Although the examples used in the text are developed out of our supervisory experiences with these students and clients, each example has been modified to preserve anonymity of people and events.

Finally, we wish to thank Decky Fiedler, Mary Beth VanBourgondien, Martha Perry, and Susie Anschell for their helpful comments on the manuscript. The clerical assistance of Peggy Jacobs, Laurie Carlson, Diane Anderson, Tsusumi Herrera, and Marlene Kerbis is also gratefully acknowledged.

J.S.Z.
R.B.
D.J.N.
I.S.D.

July, 1977

Part I
Approaching the task

1

Initial expectations

The transformation from student to professional therapist is rarely smooth or easy. Learning to be a psychotherapist forces the beginner to confront many complex
and confusing issues. Initially, many of us entered professional training with definite expectations with regard
to therapy and the role of the therapist. However, it is
often easier to imagine the rewards and gratifications of
practicing therapy than to appreciate fully the conflicts
and difficulties. In this chapter we will explore some of
the unexpected and difficult aspects of therapy that are
not often anticipated.

Many of the expectations initially held by students
change as a result of their experiences during training.
We believe that an examination of these expectations
will be a useful preparation for your training in psychotherapy. These expectations greatly influence the kinds
of problems and personal confusions students frequently
experience. It is our hope that by exploring some of these
expectations we can help you understand many of the
important issues regarding therapy, therapists, and the
people who seek therapy.

Although every person has his or her particular reasons
for deciding to become a therapist, there are some generally shared motivations among students in this field. Student and professional therapists, for instance, share a
concern for other people's welfare and a desire to be helpful in improving the quality of their lives. Often students

3

have found that helping others is personally rewarding and fulfilling, and they expect similar satisfactions from being a therapist.

In addition, many of us have selected this profession because we perceive ourselves as possessing personal characteristics that will be valuable to the practice of therapy. "Sensitive and understanding," "perceptive and insightful" are the sorts of descriptions that therapists like to apply to themselves and that others may have used to describe them. Students in this field have frequently been told that they are "good listeners"; furthermore, their advice may have been constructive and helpful to friends during periods of crisis.

An interest and curiosity about human beings and their behavior is another motive that often prompts a person to become a psychotherapist. It is this curiosity about why people think and act the way they do that often provides an impetus for developing not only a framework for understanding clients' problems, but also strategies for treatment.

Students often have other than altruistic motives for becoming therapists. Learning about therapy is frequently seen as an opportunity for students to help themselves with their own emotional problems. The practice of psychotherapy is often perceived as a way of sharing important knowledge and insights the student feels he or she has acquired. In some cases, moreover, students are attracted to becoming a therapist because of the power and privileges associated with the role.

Confusions

The expectations, personal characteristics, and motives that have drawn an individual to a therapy career may also result in a number of initial confusions and difficulties. To illustrate, the desire to be helpful is often of central importance to a beginning psychotherapist. It may result from his or her desire to be liked, to be nurturant, or to be controlling. In the extreme, these needs may produce problems in treatment. Being "helpful" may be satisfying for you as the therapist, but you may be correspondingly less responsive to the needs of your client.

For example, if the therapist is constantly more concerned and "working" harder than the client, he or she might actually hinder the process of therapy by not giving the client the opportunity to develop coping and decision-making skills. This approach by the therapist may also maintain dependent patterns of interacting that are problematic for clients in their daily social relationships.

In addition, although it is often useful to rely on your own personal experience as a guide for understanding and dealing with matters discussed by your client, it is also crucial to recognize that your own experience and personal feelings may not parallel those of your client. It is easy to assume you know what a client is feeling, based on your own experiences and reactions; however, your assumptions may be in error. Consequently, you may eliminate the possibility of understanding the unique nature of the client's dilemma. The client, believing that he or she is being understood, may consequently not explain material in the detail you would need for real understanding. Let us use as an example the client with a very conservative religious upbringing. It may be difficult for a therapist with no religious background to understand the depth and influence of religious feeling in the client's life. Missing or minimizing this point might be a serious deficit in your assessment of the client's problems and treatment.

As we've said, new therapists are likely to view and interpret their client's behavior and feelings within the framework of their own experiences. As a consequence, they may tend to regard a client's behavior as similar to what they are familiar with and disregard those aspects that fall outside their range of experience. Often the extreme or exaggerated nature of what is reported in therapy is minimized and is regarded instead as part of normal experience.

For instance, if your client did not look you in the eye at all during your initial interview, you might interpret this as a manifestation of shyness. If he or she laughed while relating apparently sad or tragic life experiences, you might call it nervous laughter. Furthermore, if the client had a history of few or no close interpersonal relationships, you might think that many people don't. In isolation each of these patterns is not that unusual, and we've probably all experienced or observed them to some degree; however, when viewed together they take on different and more serious implications.

It is easy to rely on your previous experience as the guide for therapy. What occurs in therapy is similar in many ways to what occurs frequently in conversations with our friends. That is, one may share confidences, seek and give advice, and provide support and assurances about situations or problems. This superficial similarity between therapy and friendship produces difficulties for beginning therapists who view the situations as comparable in all respects.

In actuality, a therapeutic relationship is not the same as a friendship. The client is not a friend, but a stranger who comes to you because you are labeled an expert in dealing with problems in living. The client is likely to be paying a fee in order to interact with you, and the focus in the interaction is on the client and his or her concerns, not yours. You as the therapist cannot approach the therapy situation with the same attitudes and expectations that are appropriate to a friendship.

For instance, when talking with a friend you usually have greater familiarity and knowledge of each other, so that you can gauge the response you will get to a certain type of comment. You certainly have less authority in your friendships, so that the remarks you make do not carry the weighty implications they often do with clients. Joking about a problem situation may have very different connotations for a friend than for a client. In fact, you will want to think it through very carefully before you treat lightly any concerns that a client presents.

Similarly, you may want to describe and share your own experiences when discussing a friend's problems. Therapists do not usually have this latitude and have to be careful about their use of self-disclosure. It is important to know your client extremely well before launching into a discourse about your own experiences in dealing with the situation he or she is describing.

The same is true with offering suggestions or advice. You might find that a piece of advice that has been very helpful to a friend is rebuffed by a client. Although you are likely to have an idea of how responsive your friends are to your advice, often with clients you do not have a good conception of how they respond to advice and how they view you and the role you are taking with them. Offering advice, for example, might be viewed by the client as another authority figure not understanding, telling him or her to do something. In addition, certain forms of advice giving may not be consistent with the goals of your treatment approach.

Fears

A client comes to a therapy session in obvious distress; her life is falling apart; nothing seems to be working out. All she can think of is the hopelessness of it all. She relates all her problems to you, and you try to discuss different options or views of the events. Nothing you say makes her feel better, and you cannot think of anything more to say. She sits staring silently at you.

A teen-age boy is brought to therapy by his parents. He has been engaging in delinquent behavior for several years. Recently his parents have discovered that he has been selling drugs. They are furious and can only talk about the bad things the boy has done. The boy begins shouting angrily at his parents, and they start shouting back. You are

7

confused by the fighting and unsure of how to react. At this point the parents challenge your competence to handle their problems and ask you what you are going to do about the boy.

These nightmarish situations demonstrate one of the most common fears of beginning therapists – that of being perceived as incompetent by the client. Lack of skill is often an all too obvious fact to the novice. This, coupled with the ambiguity and unclearness of the criteria for adequate performance as a therapist, heightens the self-criticism and doubt bred initially by the newness of the role.

Some students react to the fears of being perceived as incompetent by attempting to bluff their way through the session by "acting like a therapist" (e.g., by acting distant, authoritative, and uncommunicative). Others may reveal their insecurity or lack of knowledge to the client and try to promote a buddy relationship. It is often helpful to remember that two of the most common obstacles to learning to be a therapist result from preconceptions students may have with regard to how they should appear and from the fear of looking incompetent.

Most new therapists find it difficult to accept the fact that they do not need to provide an answer for every question, that they do not have to respond immediately to everything the client presents. It is quite legitimate, even wise, to take time to think about your response to an issue and consult with your supervisor about it. It's even quite acceptable to tell your client that you'd like to think about an issue a while before responding.

Students also often hesitate to admit their fears and frustrations about their performance to other students and to supervisors in the mistaken belief that everyone else is doing better than they. Many years of schooling have left students with severe fears of negative evaluation and a sense of competition with peers. Rather than being able to take solace in the fact that others experience similar problems, they are often left isolated and fearful.

8

The fears of failure and poor evaluation often produce a severe conflict for the beginning psychotherapist in regard to supervision. He or she may be reluctant to admit ignorance or uncertainty about how to proceed with a case because of concern about negative evaluation. At those times it is easier to relate what is succeeding with a client than it is to discuss the difficulties and uncertainty you are experiencing. In our supervision of students we find that at times they interpret the demands on them as a "double-bind" situation; that is, they are asked to be open and honest about their difficulties, but are simultaneously evaluated by supervisors on the number and extent of these difficulties. Conflicts such as these need to be worked out in individual supervisory and evaluative relationships; however, they illustrate the complicated nature of the psychotherapy teaching process.

Related to the fear of looking bad to clients, supervisors, and peers is the fear of losing the client. Every client terminates therapy sooner or later, and some terminate it prematurely. Beginning therapists fear that an untimely termination indicates their failure as a therapist. This is a one-sided and frequently overly optimistic view of therapy. The process of reaching solutions for emotional problems is much more of a mutual responsibility, shared by the client and therapist, than students may initially understand.

This former line of reasoning implies that the only determining factor for a client's continuing or terminating therapy is his or her interaction with the therapist. Although the impact of the therapist should not be minimized, this view does not take into consideration the many other factors that influence the decisions an individual might make about terminating therapy. At times a therapist may lose perspective on the fact that therapy is only a part of the client's life and that monetary, interpersonal, or environmental factors may influence both the problems a person is experiencing and decisions regarding therapy.

9

Similarly, students are likely to feel uncomfortable with what seems to be a very slow rate of progress and to feel responsible for producing changes faster. There is a frequent desire to see change occur immediately. Students often complain, "The client isn't getting any better," or, "Nothing is changing with this client." Whether or not progress is being made is not always obvious. A beginner finds it very difficult to estimate what an acceptable rate of progress is, because of a lack of experience with the long-term progress of a number of clients.

This brief examination of some common motives, confusions, and fears is intended to help you feel more comfortable about dealing with these situations when they arise during your training. They involve issues with which therapists must grapple throughout their careers. The questions of responsibility, personal motivations, most effective type of interaction with clients, self-doubts, and treatment procedures seem never to be definitively answered. You, like all other therapists, are likely to be constantly reevaluating and changing your opinions on these matters.

2

Professional responsibilities

Ethical and legal issues

Generally, the highest priority for you as a student therapist is your progress in developing clinical skills: what to do with a client and how to do it most effectively. The legal and ethical matters that will assume considerable importance when you become involved in clinical practice are often neglected during this learning process. It has been our experience that students enter training without having given much thought to the professional aspects of their work. However, early consideration of these issues is important, because they enter into the decisions you will make with clients from your initial contacts. The question of confidentiality, for example, is a fundamental issue that both you and the client will probably discuss in your first interview.

Some of the other perplexing questions students face are the following: "What are my legal and ethical responsibilities toward a client?" "What are my obligations to society?" "What are my services worth?" "Under what circumstances may I or must I violate confidentiality?" We've written this chapter to acquaint you with some of the issues these questions involve. It is hoped that our discussion will be of help to you in answering them.

Professional responsibility and liability. We've found that beginning students often experience discomfort about seeing clients during practicum work because they are insecure about their limited skills. This situation necessarily arises because the only way to develop clinical skills is through actual experience. You will need to practice first in order to become accomplished at therapy. There is ample legal and public recognition of the need for practicum training in our professions; thus, most laws that control professional clinical practice provide for students to do work in training settings under the supervision of qualified clinicians. The legal or social sanction for students to do therapy derives from the public sanction of the training facility and supervisors. In fact, most mental health professionals practice under some legal or professional accreditation. State laws also provide for the titling of people in training. You will probably find it necessary to familiarize yourself with the state laws or professional association guidelines pertinent to your field.

During your practicum experiences, then, you are actually operating under the licensure or certification of your supervisors. Even though you have the primary responsibility for your clients, treatment is legally under their control and direction. The supervisor must assume professional and legal responsibility, including liability for inadequate or negligent treatment.

This issue of responsibility has implications for how you relate to your supervisors. Many students are insecure about their own judgment and skills and rely heavily on their supervisors for direct suggestions for action. Others, particularly as they gain experience, prefer to operate fairly autonomously. Supervisors also differ tremendously in their tolerance for independence on the part of students. In any event, from a legal point of view you will need to keep your supervisor well informed about your case. Keeping your supervisor informed provides protection for you, your client, and the supervisor.

Maintaining adequate records increases this protection, particularly in a training clinic setting. Session-by-session note taking provides vital information to a staff member who may have to handle a case in your absence or after you have finished with a client and left the program. In addition to giving others necessary information, note keeping gives you perspective on the progress of your client over the course of therapy.

Written records also play an important role when negligent or unprofessional behavior is being investigated. In many instances, particularly in a legal dispute, one's recollection of case material may not be sufficient. Courts tend to downgrade evidence about care that is not substantiated with session-by-session record keeping. For example, in the investigation of a client's suicide a verbal report that you recommended hospitalization would not carry the same weight as a written record.

Confidentiality. From the very first session students and clients are concerned about the issues of confidentiality involved in their therapeutic interactions. It is not uncommon for a client to begin the initial interview by asking about the confidentiality of the information revealed during therapy hours. Your clients may be involved in life situations that do not sanction psychotherapy, and they may fear negative consequences if their confidentiality is violated. Possible destructive consequences include legal liability, divorce, or loss of employment.

The state laws covering mental health professions usually make some provision for the confidentiality of information revealed in therapy hours. It is important that you understand that the legal privilege is extended to the client, not the therapist. This means that no information regarding clients may be disclosed without their written permission. You and the clinic in which you are working are legally liable if you reveal any information about a client without his or her written consent. Again, the legalities of confidentiality differ from state to state, and you will want to learn the specifics in your own area.

However, the usual rule is that one must not disclose information to anyone, even a spouse, parent, or employer, whatever the intent, except in very special situations. For example, evidence of child abuse has sometimes been excluded from the confidentiality privilege, and you may be required legally to report an incident of this type told to you by a client. This legal constraint may present a serious ethical dilemma for you when a client has come to you for help with problems in this area.

As illustrated in this example, privileged communication may pose ethical difficulties for a therapist. For instance, what about maintaining confidentiality in cases of murder, serious felonies, or an imminent suicide? Your ethical concerns for your clients or those around them might demand that you intervene, break confidentiality, and risk civil liability. The legal issues regarding confidentiality in these gray areas are presently unclear, and these questions have no easy answers.

There are some other special confidentiality issues and problems that will arise, because of supervision requirements, while you are in training. You will be called on to explain to your clients that others, who are supervising you, have access to their confidential information and to explain why this is so. In addition, many clinics routinely use audio and video taping as a tool in supervision. You and your clients may find the exposure and scrutiny imposed by taping to be disturbing. We encourage our students to discuss such training requirements openly with clients in a matter-of-fact way. Our experience indicates that the more directly their concerns are discussed, the easier it is for both therapists and clients to overcome their self-consciousness at being observed by supervisors or fellow students.

In any event, it is essential that clients be aware of the implications of a training setting and the extent to which information is shared among staff members. Training situations independently introduce many complicated issues to the therapy relationship; you will need to consider these matters thoughtfully, with an understanding of the rights of the client.

Presenting yourself as a professional

Students in training are often concerned about how they should introduce themselves, how important their style of dress is, and a variety of other issues about meeting clients for the first time. We've found certain considerations useful in helping students deal with these concerns.

A client seeking therapy arrives with a set of expectations about the clinic and the practitioner. These expectations need to be considered by the therapist in determining how he or she acts and relates to the client. Generally, people expect a therapist to be knowledgeable and competent to deal with their problems in what is established culturally as a professional manner. A client's first impressions about competency are influenced by the physical environment of the clinic, the reception he or she receives, and the appearance and manner of the therapist.

At the time of the initial contact you will not know the client's expectations, biases, or sensitivities. We think it is wise to dress fairly conservatively, to avoid offending a client or creating unnecessary negative expectations. In the typical clinic or hospital setting, for example, wearing exceptionally casual clothing may be viewed by a client as a sign of indifference, despite your actual level of concern. When there is very little else to base them on, the client's impressions regarding competence and potential helpfulness will likely be set by these kinds of initial impressions.

Greeting a client at the first interview is a matter of some consternation for people in training. "How should I present myself?" students often ask. We suggest that the best practice is to use a title descriptive of their role, such as psychological intern, resident, medical student, or graduate student in training. Whether to present yourself by first, last, or both names is also somewhat of a dilemma. Since this is the first interview, you are likely to convey the least "surplus meaning" by referring to your-

15

self as Dr., Mr., or Ms. or by using your full name. The same holds true for calling the client by his or her full name.

Related to the questions about dress and presentation is the student's concern about professional credibility. Many students have difficulty conveying both that their work is being supervised and monitored and that, nevertheless, they are themselves competent and confident. For some students these two matters seem to be contradictory. It is our experience that no one is served by the student therapist indulging in labored honesty about his or her shortcomings, deficiencies, or lack of experience. Yet sometimes one's feelings of insecurity may make that alternative appear attractive. For instance, a client may well ask, "Have you ever helped someone like me before?" and the likelihood is that you haven't. It is reasonable in such a situation to emphasize that you have skills that can be of help, that members of the clinic staff have had experience with similar problems, and that you will draw on that experience as necessary. Obviously, as a student in training you are not expected to be fully experienced and skilled. However, you have a responsibility to be aware of situations that surpass your present competencies and to seek out supervisory support in these instances.

In this section we've dealt with issues and concerns that are critical to the student as he or she begins to see clients in psychotherapy. Making the transition from student to psychotherapist involves tremendous personal and professional changes and is often a very confusing experience. Many of the questions discussed here have no right or wrong answers for all situations or all individuals. Our purpose has been more to encourage you to continue to think about them than to provide you with solutions.

Part II

First client contact and assessment

3

Preparations

Although clinics vary considerably with regard to the type and amount of information provided to the therapist, there is usually an opportunity to learn something about an incoming client prior to his or her arrival. In some settings the regular full-time staff will conduct the initial treatment evaluations and assign student therapists afterward. In other settings the client's name is the only information requested prior to the first interview and it is up to you to gather sufficient information to evaluate the client's problems and develop a treatment plan. This chapter focuses on how to prepare for your first contact with a client, regardless of the amount of prior information you have as a basis for your planning. It will also alert you to some sources of information you may not have considered.

Planning your initial strategy ahead of time, with a supervisor, if possible, is a valuable ingredient in conducting an effective interview and learning to be a therapist. Beginners find it particularly difficult to "think on their feet"; they tend to be easily distracted or overwhelmed by the unexpected. Student therapists can maximize their initial effectiveness and rapport with a client by anticipating the particular sensitivities of the person they are interviewing and the areas about which he or she may have difficulty talking. Thoughtful preparation around these issues may make the difference between an initial interview that sets the stage for successful treatment and one that ends with the client being uncertain about returning.

Information gathering

There are two steps in the process of preparing for your first interview. The first is collecting and examining the information available to you from what the client has stated in the application materials, how he or she behaved while applying, and what his or her experience was like with your clinic. The second step involves speculating about the significance of this information and planning mini-strategies that will help you conduct your interview.

Rather than prejudging someone before gathering all the information, your job as therapist is to hypothesize about behavior, sensitivities, and possible problem areas for the client. Using these hypotheses you can develop an interview strategy that will be aimed at maximizing the client's comfort and your efficiency in gathering information. However, your hypotheses should be flexible and tentative and open to confirmation or rejection on the basis of further experience with the client.

Information from the application form. Many clinical settings request biographical information, such as age, educational level, working status and occupation, marital and living situation, referral source, and previous therapists as part of their client application material. Discrepancies within this information may alert you to potential sources of problems.

> A twenty-seven-year-old male client's application indicated that he had completed some work toward a graduate degree, had a work history that included teaching and garbage collecting, and was currently employed as a janitor. This information alerted the interviewer to possible conflict in the work area.

20

Keep in mind, however, that inconsistencies may not necessarily reflect current difficulties; however, an obvious discrepancy is always worth investigating.

A client's responses to questions about marital status, family, and living situation may alert you to other problems. This information also provides some basic picture of this person's life within which to place and assess further information you gather. Knowledge about the client's living situation may give you very useful information about sources of support or *lack* of support that may affect the treatment approach you choose. Although one's living situation may not be the primary source of conflict, it is always useful for the therapist to make an assessment of the client's current life situation and its possible impact.

Some noteworthy examples include the sixteen-year-old girl who is living alone and is legally independent from her parents, the single forty-year-old man who is living at home with his widowed mother, or the man who reports being married and living without his wife but with their two children. In the case of the teen-age girl living alone, for example, you would certainly want to know more about how this living situation was established and what it means in terms of other adult influences and possible supports in her life.

The source by which a client is referred may also be a significant factor. Information about the type of people who usually reach a given referral source, the individuals typically referred to other clinics and why, and the way a referral is usually conducted can all be valuable. This information gives you some idea about the type of experiences your client may have had prior to contacting you. It is important to remember, however, that each person's experience with a given referral source will be different to some extent; prior information should be used only to formulate hypotheses, not to prejudice your view of your client.

A referral coming from within the court system, for

instance, may indicate that the client has been coerced into seeking treatment and that he or she may be resistive to therapy. Another example is the client who has been referred by a large social service agency. Such an individual may have had to go through a lot of red tape, which may have caused him or her to be impatient with the system, and you may bear the brunt of these frustrations.

Similarly, clients who have seen six or seven previous therapists are possibly searching for some particular answer to their problems that you, like the others, may not be able to provide. A long history of contact with mental health professionals could also indicate a chronic difficulty in dealing with problems in living. On the other hand, a client who has been in therapy one or two times previously may have positive expectations for change that will make future success more likely. You can be fairly confident that whether a client's previous experience in therapy was positive or negative, prior exposure to a mental health professional will have an effect on the client's expectations for current treatment.

Quite often clinics also ask the new client to state his or her reason for seeking therapy. However, you may find that the problem the client states on the application form is not always the primary issue of concern. Applicants often find their way into treatment by expressing acceptable problems, such as "trouble concentrating on school work," to cover less acceptable ones, such as "fear of going crazy." Similarly, be alert to people who enter therapy requesting treatment approaches that are current in the media or claiming problems that are in vogue, such as in the example of assertive training that follows. Although these may be valid reasons for seeking help, they also may be masking another sort of problem that is primary but more difficult for the individual to recognize. Some examples:

> The parents of a five-year-old child applied for therapy for their son because of difficulties his teacher reported in controlling him in kindergarten. However, a thorough

22

evaluation of the situation revealed that the parents were having severe marital difficulties and were in conflict about discipline methods for the child.

A married forty-year-old woman applied for assertiveness training, complaining that she needed those skills in her work situation; however, it also became clear during the interview that her marriage to a strong-willed, controlling man was actually her major source of concern. She was unwilling to question her marriage because of her fears of being lonely and unable to support herself and two children.

In addition to examining the content of the information provided by the client, it is useful to pay attention to other aspects of the client's reasons, style, or appearance of the application materials that are unusual in any way. Such deviations are often extremely informative. For example, idiosyncratic or unique wording on the application form may alert you to a client's possible confusion or difficulty in thought and verbal expression.

There are a variety of peculiarities that you may encounter in reading application forms. Some applicants say as little as they can possibly get away with while still providing the information requested. Such people may be more revealing when actually being interviewed, but they are more likely to be equally reticent about providing information in person. A prime reason may be suspiciousness, but other possibilities are shyness, shame, lack of verbal skills, or confusion and disorganization. The interviewer in this situation should try to draw the client out as much as possible in order to develop some hypotheses about what is behind the reticence.

The omission of information that has been requested can also be noteworthy; it may indicate that the client is suspicious, fearful of exposure, or unwilling to reveal his or her private affairs. Attention to the content of the omissions may point to particularly sensitive areas for the client. Such cues can be used as a guide in structuring the interview. When crucial information, such as marital status or occupation, is omitted, you will need to inquire about it. It is important to do so, however, in a manner that is not overly abrupt or damaging to your developing rapport with the client. This may require you to postpone such questions until a second interview so that both you and your client are somewhat more at ease and prepared to deal with potentially sensitive topics. With increased experience you will gain a sense of proper timing for such an inquiry.

Skimpily answered application forms are commonly encountered, but you will probably also run across the other extreme. Some potential clients write at great length in response to application questions, providing specifics in exceptional detail. This situation brings two possibilities to mind: first, that the individual is highly disturbed, with loose, disorganized thinking; and second, that he or she is highly perfectionistic and obsessive. In these cases control is likely to be an issue in the interview. Some people may be prepared to offer you a well-rehearsed script elaborating on their problems; others may be too disorganized to offer a coherent explanation of why they are seeking help. With either type of client, considerable structuring of the interview will probably be necessary to collect the information you need in order to develop a treatment plan. For the obsessive type of individual you may need to be firm and directive; the disorganized person may benefit from structuring of a more supportive, reassuring, and reflecting nature. A disturbed, disorganized person may also require more closure and direction when you end the interview.

Vague replies to application questions are also revealing; a client's indirect or nonspecific answers may reflect a difficulty in defining problems.

> A young man entered therapy because of feelings of sexual inadequacy. However, it was difficult to ascertain the specifics of his sex life. After much specific questioning it became clear that the problem was primarily his partner's inability to have orgasm during intercourse. Treatment in-

volved quite a different approach from that which the therapist had anticipated on the basis of the client's initial statement.

Clients who persist in giving general answers to questions require lengthy and sometimes tedious pursuit by the interviewer. If you don't set out very firmly to do this, you may end up with only vague information about the client's problems. Such a situation could easily result in serious misperceptions on your part.

Having the application materials with you during the interview can often be helpful in reminding you of lines of questioning you want to follow. Having this prior information can be very useful in your planning. However, not all clinical settings request such materials; some clinics, such as college counseling centers, do not ask their applicants for much in the way of prior written information. Usually these settings serve a clientele that might be alienated by having to fill out forms in an impersonal manner. If you work in such a setting you will need to rely on the following, more informal sources of information.

The client's behavior. The client's manner and actions during the application process provide considerable information. We find it useful to look at the person's approach to the application for therapy as a sample of the client's behavior in other life situations.

His or her telephone manner, style of dress, arrival time, cancellations, behavior toward secretarial personnel, attitude toward payment of fees, and behavior in the waiting room are all rich informational sources. The client has probably had contact with someone in your clinic about his or her request for therapy. Clinic staff are generally trained and experienced in picking up nuances of behavior that may reflect a client's personality style, attitude toward treatment, or problem areas. We strongly recommend that you check out all informal sources of knowledge within the clinic in order to maximize the comfort and effectiveness of your first interview. This information is important but should be used in conjunction with other information about the client.

People with interpersonal problems are likely to reveal various aspects of their difficulties when applying to your clinic. Hostility, shyness, impatience, suspiciousness, and lack of social skills may be expressed toward the secretary or screening person during the first telephone call or visit to the clinic. You may be alerted to the possibility that a client, for instance, is concerned with confidentiality and likely to be suspicious. In such a case you can plan ahead to ensure that you attend particularly to these concerns. Likewise, your strategy with a person who has been angry and quietly sullen with the receptionist will differ from that with a client whose silences appear to reflect painful shyness. Whereas a quietly shy person might welcome additional structure and directiveness from you, an angry client may be further antagonized by control imposed by the interviewer.

A person's willingness to provide information requested by the secretary may give you some notion of how difficult it will be to elicit private or personal information during the interview. On the other hand, you may find that a person is impatient and distant toward the secretary but exceedingly agreeable with you.

The following are some examples of cases worth noting:

Although the secretary has explained the clinic procedures thoroughly to the client, he has continued to call daily about forgotten details.

A client requests therapy for marital difficulties but is extremely insistent that the clinic staff not return his call when his wife might be at home.

A client is angry about having to pay a fee and insists on knowing ahead of time what he is going to get for his money.

The receptionist noted that the client, while waiting for his appointment, would not look at anyone else in the office and averted his eyes when spoken to.

Many different interpretations may be developed with the preceding examples, depending on the other knowledge you have about the client. Difficulties in making and keeping appointments may call into question the client's motivation for treatment. However, other reasons may be operating; for instance, the client's lack of assertiveness may be preventing him or her from asking for time off from work to come in for therapy appointments. Although such information about a client can be valuable, its meaning varies, depending on the context of that individual's experience. Once again, your job at this point is to form hypotheses, not to become wedded to any specific assumptions about the reasons for a client's behavior.

The client's experiences. The client's previous contact with your clinic may have a profound effect on his or her attitude and manner when you first meet. For example, knowing how long the client has been on the clinic's waiting list before being interviewed is a critical piece of information. If the waiting period has been long, it is possible that the immediate problems are resolved; people typically apply for therapy during a crisis, which often is resolved in some way within several weeks. For some people the simple act of applying for treatment provides them with a sense of relief and resolution. For others the problems grow to the extent that they feel compelled to make some major life change, such as quitting a job or separating from their spouse, in order to resolve the problem. In any event, it is extremely unlikely that the situation has remained the same. The client's feelings about having to wait an extended period may also emerge during your first contact, and you should be prepared to respond to them.

A client's experiences in your clinic waiting room may also be powerful determinants of how he or she will react to you at the first interview. For example:

A client has been in the waiting room and has seen another client leave looking very upset.

27

The secretary was not informed of the client's appointment. The client was told that he or she was not expected.

A client inadvertently overheard a group of clinic staff joking about another person, possibly a client.

The client's attitude toward you, your clinic, his or her problems, and therapy in general may be seriously affected by these kinds of experiences. It is important for you to be alert to what is happening to your client *before* you bring him or her into the interview room. Following is a particularly dramatic example of the importance of such experiences: While waiting for his initial interview, a young Asian American college student encountered an Asian graduate student in the clinic. As his interviewer soon learned, his personal and cultural reticence about seeking therapy was greatly exacerbated by meeting another person of his own ethnic group with whom he had previously worked as a research assistant. If the therapist had not been aware of the encounter and sensitive to its implications, the client probably never would have returned. By mentioning this event early in the session and questioning the client about his reaction to it, the therapist was able to reassure the client that his confidentiality would be respected.

In summary, there are a number of formal and informal methods of gaining some knowledge about a client before you actually sit down with him or her in the initial interview. The value of this information comes not from the help it gives you in reaching some specific judgment about this person prior to meeting him or her, but from the help it gives in forming some hypotheses about your client that will guide your structuring of the interview. You must be prepared to have many of your hypotheses disproved; to cling too firmly to your hypotheses can lead to gross misinterpretations of a client's behavior. It is equally important to be prepared to alter your style of dealing with a client in response to new information you will learn during the interview. Impressions based on prior experience with an individual may suggest an approach that is not the most productive in the context of a structured interview. Flexibility on your part is essential.

As your personal field of experience broadens, you will become increasingly sensitive to significant informational sources and to integrating the bits and pieces of knowledge about a client into a meaningful picture. The systematic, step-by-step examination of information that we have outlined for you in this chapter is a training device for the beginner. As you gain experience these preparations become considerably shortened and semiautomatic.

4

The initial interview

At first, beginning therapists view initial interviewing as merely gathering information on the problem that brings the client to therapy. After completing their first interview, however, beginners frequently feel overwhelmed and bewildered by the subtle and complex skills required. Conducting an effective initial interview involves mastering two skills: first, establishing a comfortable, accepting atmosphere that allows the client to communicate freely; second, gathering the necessary information regarding the client's problems so that you can make an adequate assessment of the situation and develop an appropriate treatment plan.

We cannot provide you with written guidelines covering all the various situations you will encounter in your interviewing. This is a major reason why supervision is such a crucial aspect of the therapeutic learning process. Each client will present you with different challenges, and each new interviewing situation must be approached with flexibility. We find that students frequently forget that exceptions are almost always the rule in clinical practice. Although each interview will call for a slightly different course of action, we will offer some general suggestions about initial interviewing that have been useful to beginners.

The first interview: what to expect

The first interview is typically a frightening situation for both the client and the beginning therapist. It is a time of mutual evaluation, one in which both of you may well be extremely concerned about what the *other* thinks.

Clients are usually uneasy about asking a professional for help, nearly as anxious about this prospect as they are about the problems themselves. They enter the initial interview with a multitude of fears and expectations, many of which are quite exaggerated. Your client may be afraid of being thought of as "crazy" or of being seen as weak or dependent. He or she is usually unsure about what is expected and may be afraid to reveal highly personal and possibly damaging information to a stranger. In training settings clients may wonder in addition about the competence of the therapist and if their problems are too serious or shocking for a beginner.

To counterbalance some of these overwhelming fears, a client may develop expectations about the benefits of therapy and the powers of the therapist that are quite unrealistic. Some clients believe that the therapist knows their thoughts. They may expect that the therapist has the power magically to eradicate their problems, anticipating that therapy will involve only a few short sessions. Unfortunately, the expectations for benefit must sometimes be quite grandiose to offset the fears involved.

The fears and expectations your client brings to the initial sessions can have a powerful effect on you. The scope of the problems may increase your feeling of being inadequate and ignorant and at the same time may add to the pressure you already feel to provide understanding and help. The demand to do something becomes a major concern that leads the student to give advice, reassurance, or a plan of action prematurely.

In addition to responding to the perceptions of the client, every therapist experiences his or her own personal anxieties about the initial interview. Your own fears about appearing incompetent; failing to control the interview; not knowing what to say; or encountering an uncooperative, silent, or, worse yet, hostile client may severely interfere with the task at hand. In combination

31

with the client's concerns, the anxiety in the initial interviewing room can disturb the exchange of information considerably. You need to have your own anxieties reasonably well in hand in order to be able both to alleviate the client's fears and to conduct a productive information-gathering session.

Some suggestions for putting yourself at ease

Devising the seating arrangement and acquainting yourself with the physical layout of the room in advance of the session may help you feel more comfortable when first meeting your client. Taking charge of the social mechanics of the interview may also enhance your feelings of control and confidence. For example, identifying and introducing yourself without apologies, firmly directing the client to the interview room, and specifying the seat he or she is to take often provide the interviewer with an increased sense of confidence and comfort in the professional role.

Although we do not recommend note taking during interviews as a routine practice, it may serve to allay anxiety about what to do initially. Some individuals can take notes quite unobtrusively without interfering with the flow of the conversation; others, however, find it a distraction rather than an aid. For note taking to be helpful you must be able to listen to the client's conversation closely enough to be able to follow up important comments while at the same time jotting down pertinent facts. This is a fairly difficult task, one that beginners are often unable to carry off smoothly and effectively.

We often reassure students by making them aware of their options. For example, they needn't have an answer to every question the client asks. It is also helpful to keep in mind that almost everything you say is reparable. You'll have other opportunities to ask questions you've forgotten or to clarify a confused point. Silence is not necessarily bad. It may give the client a chance to reflect or m⸤y encourage him or her to expand on a topic. Expressing bewilderment when something appears to be confusing is often quite appropriate. Even leaving the room to consult with a supervisor may be called for in some emergency situations. When you are in doubt about what direction to pursue in an interview, you can wait for the client to continue, repeat yourself, or ask for further elaboration. Every therapist has had a momentary lapse of memory and has forgotten the reason why a client has come in for help. One need not panic; gentle inquiry will soon jog your memory.

Only increased experience will produce a solid sense of confidence and competence as a therapist; however, some of these preparations will assist beginners in feeling more at ease. Discussing what to expect from a particular client with supervisors or colleagues can often be reassuring, unless of course you become so wedded to your expectations that you are not able to cope with a different reality that the client may present.

Conducting the initial interview

As we have pointed out in the second chapter, there are certain practical considerations that must be addressed with a client seeking help in a training clinic. For example, the supervision or taping requirements must be explained and agreed on. In addition, it is important that the client understand how the intake procedure works and what part the initial interview plays in it. After covering these points, the therapist might ask one of the following questions to begin the interview: "What brings you here?" or, "How may I be of help?"

The client will usually begin talking about some aspect of his or her difficulties, and the therapist can gently guide the client's account to clarify and expand his or her understanding. This is the ideal situation, but unfortunately you may not encounter ideal interviewees in your training. Some clients seem to want to discuss other people and their problems, give descriptive history, provide excessive details, or discuss a variety of topics not connected to their need for therapy. Therapists must sometimes exert considerable control and directiveness in order to keep the client talking about the problem areas. Following are some examples of such directive comments:

"I'd like to get back to your major concerns."

"How does this relate to the problems that bring you to the clinic?"

"I'm confused. I think I need to know more about your current problems before I can help you."

"I would like to know something about your upbringing, but first I'd like to understand . . . more fully."

"I'm wondering if it wouldn't be more productive to focus on your current situation for the time being."

"I think I'll need to know more about your goals for therapy before I can help you."

Gathering the relevant information about the client and his or her behaviors may be a straightforward or an exceedingly complicated matter. Some clients require little prompting from you to elicit elaboration or clarification and themselves provide direction as to the areas to pursue. When you have covered an area to your satisfaction, you can change to another topic by making one of the following transition statements:

"Besides knowing about the problem area, I would also like to know something about other aspects of your life."

"I think I understand why you've come here. Now I'd like to know something about your current life situation."

"I also would like to know something about your background and family."

Some clients will come to you not knowing why they are upset; they may be tearful and disorganized or fearful and silent. In these more difficult situations you may need to calm the person by demonstrating your understanding, concern, and acceptance and by providing some structure before attempting to learn about the specific problems that bring him or her to you. For example:

> A young woman came to her initial interview and proceeded to cry uncontrollably, unable to communicate clearly. She was concerned about "breaking down" and this thought preoccupied her to the exclusion of all else. She claimed not to know why she was upset. The woman calmed down only after considerable reassurance from the therapist that there was nothing wrong with showing her feelings by crying. Through gradually asking questions about events of her day, the therapist and client discovered that an interaction with a critical instructor had been the initial precipitating event.

Clients often begin to discuss their problems and are unable to continue because the experience of simply telling another person what troubles them is itself extremely upsetting. It is common for a client to cry at the very onset of the interview, and something you might expect. At such times it is best to provide understanding, support, and acceptance and not to try to force the information gathering until the client has collected himself or herself. If this pattern continues throughout the interview, one may have to adopt the strategy of "pushing on."

Other clients will bring with them special concerns or agendas that may interfere with gathering information in the interview. For example:

> A client begins the interview by recounting his negative feelings about the receptionist in the clinic and his very mixed feelings about talking to you. He insists that he was "reaching out for help" but that the attitudes of the professionals he had encountered have been anything but helpful, and that he did not know if he wanted to tell you anything at all.

In dealing with such a situation, the therapist communicated his respect for the client's feelings and a concern about what the client's prior experiences had been that had resulted in such negative feelings. Again, it was crucial for the interviewer not to try to force any self-disclosure until the client felt ready. In this case, when the client realized that his feelings were being treated respectfully, he was willing to talk more about his depression resulting from feeling incompetent at work. He apparently needed demonstration of the respect of the therapist before allowing himself any signs of "weakness."

Dealing with the client's anxiety. Students frequently see the task as one of making the client as comfortable as possible. You may have a friendly, warm interaction with the client that avoids all anxiety-provoking subjects yet succeeds in gathering very little information about the client's problems. We propose the notion of "optimum" anxiety – that is, aiming for a state where the client is not overwhelmed or paralyzed by excessive anxiety but sufficiently uncomfortable to demonstrate his or her coping skills and emotionality. You should try to strike a balance between sufficient probing of sensitive areas and attempts to keep the client's anxiety within manageable limits.

A good interviewer is sensitive to both verbal and non-verbal signs of discomfort on the part of the client, inquires about their meaning, and directly reassures the client about his or her concerns, if this is possible and appropriate.

For example, some of the following statements can be reassuring:

"People are often concerned about seeking professional help."

"I'm glad you came to see me; you seem to be very concerned about these problems, and this is a first step in doing something about them."

"It takes a good deal of courage to talk about such private matters to someone you don't know."

By bringing these concerns out in the open for discussion you will convey to the client that his or her feelings are reasonable and understandable. It's important to establish your role as an accepting, concerned, supportive individual whose job is to help the client communicate the nature of the difficulty accurately.

There are some other ways of assisting the client. For example, clearly specifying the kinds of information you want may reduce his or her anxiety considerably. Making your transitions from one topic area to another smooth and explicit will also be helpful. Clarifying and summarizing what you have heard may reassure the client that he or she is communicating something understandable. An initial information-gathering interview can in itself be therapeutic by helping the client clarify his or her confusions about what is happening.

Ideally, you will want your client to leave the first interview with an increased sense of clarity and direction. For many individuals, who are overwhelmed by anxiety and confusion, your understanding and clarification can be relieving. Telling a sympathetic, trained listener about a troublesome situation may force structure on the problems that may make them seem less overwhelming.

Following are examples of clarifying statements you may wish to make:

"Let me be sure I understand. . . . "

"I'm getting the impression that you're most upset about. . . . "

"I think I understand what you're saying." (But don't say it if you *don't* understand.)

"I'm confused about this last point. Can you clarify it?"

Some clients will come to the interview quite anxious and you may wish to engage initially in some limited small talk to put the client at ease. This tactic may also build anxiety, however, for the client who wants to "get everything out in the open." If you think the client is uncomfortable when you look directly at him or her, look away from time to time. If you think his or her level of anxiety about the interview is becoming overwhelming, change the subject, change your approach, slow down or speed up, or even end the session early. Although you may not get the information you need that particular session, you will maximize the possibility that the client will return the next time.

If your client is sitting in what looks to be an uncomfortable, tense position, if he or she is restless or constantly looking away, avoiding eye contact, blocking, or being evasive, you may speculate that anxiety is interfering with your interview. These speculations can be shared and checked out with the client, for example, by saying, "You seem tense." Sometimes, however, the client will be unable or unwilling to admit to feelings of discomfort. Your own frustration, bewilderment, and tension may also be valuable clues to indicate that you might profit from either discussing them with the client or altering your interviewing style or the topic being discussed.

One cautionary note: From time to time you may encounter clients who are apparently in no distress. You may have difficulty ascertaining the problem that brings them to therapy. In such instances the approach of choice may be to encourage the client to feel *anxious*. For example, you might express bewilderment about why he or she came in for help. Or you might pursue a sensitive area of questioning in depth until you elicit some evidence of discomfort. By doing so you may be able to determine the areas of difficulty causing stress for the client. This tactic is best left to an experienced therapist, however, or to a situation in which you are closely supervised.

Content of the first interview

The central concern of a therapist in an initial interview will be the client's presenting problem. Beginners are often satisfied with a brief statement of why the client has sought help. However, it is often a very involved issue. You will need to understand the development of the problems and the reason the client has decided to seek help at this particular time. In addition, you need to make an assessment of any dangers or immediate crises the client is facing. This information is crucial in some cases and may dictate that some immediate action, such as hospitalization, needs to be taken. This topic is covered thoroughly in a later chapter.

To assess the problem adequately you must also evaluate your client's emotional response to the difficulties. There are two components to this process: the client's verbal self-report and your observations of his or her emotional state or mood. In addition, you must thoroughly understand the client's current life situation and how it interacts with the presenting problems. Finally, it is important to determine what the client wants and expects in the way of help for these problems.

A certain amount of background information is important to assessing the severity of the problems, evaluating the client's coping skills, and understanding the development of the problems. Depending on the amount of time available, it is useful to gather some information about the patient's family, social, and medical background and any previous therapy contacts. One could easily spend five or six hours collecting information, but rarely is there adequate time for such thoroughness.

It is most important, given limited time, to acquire a detailed and thorough account of the patient's *current* problems as he or she sees them. We usually suggest that therapists begin with a fairly general query, such as, "Tell me about the problems you and your wife have been having." This gives the client the opportunity to begin with what seems most salient. From then on the therapist asks more and more specific questions until the situation becomes clear on both an emotional and behavioral level. Each area that the client brings up may be pursued in that way, from the general to the specific.

At the beginning of your training you will probably

need to make as broad-based an assessment of the client and his life as the time will allow, because you will not have acquired enough experience to develop hypotheses that will more efficiently guide your questioning. As your experience accumulates, you will become alert to verbal and nonverbal cues from the client that will suggest possible problem areas. For example, if a client shows increased signs of anxiety in discussing a topic, if contradictions are apparent to you within an area, or if the client's speech pattern, intonation, and rate of speech change while responding to a question, these might suggest conflict or difficulty that you might want to explore further. Discussing the interview with your supervisor will help alert you to these clues, but until your experience base is fairly broad it is useful to cover all areas as thoroughly as time allows.

Ending the interview

In their anxiety about doing a "good job," students may forget that the initial interview may be a very critical event for the client. This might be the first time he or she has ever revealed these problems to another person and the client may have important reactions to doing so. Clients are often concerned about the impression they've made, whether they've made good use of the therapist's time, whether they can be helped, and what's going to happen *now*.

It is important to keep track of the time to allow an opportunity to address these concerns at the end of the interview. In doing this, don't interrupt your client in the middle of an upsetting discussion; it is best to continue until the client is calmer, if possible.

At the end of the session it is useful for the therapist to summarize the concerns expressed by the client and to see if that coincides with the client's perceptions. Although it is unlikely that you will feel prepared to offer the client an assessment of the problems at this point, some general feedback is often very reassuring. For example, you might say, "It is evident that you are very concerned about these issues and that they are causing a good deal of difficulty in your life," or, "It is clear that you don't know what to do about these problems and that seeking some assistance is a wise move."

Finally, you should specify the next step in the intake process, such as an additional interviewing or feedback session, and when the client may expect this to occur. The client will have a better feeling of closure if he or she has had a chance to correct any of the therapist's misperceptions, make any additions, and ask any questions he or she may have.

Common mistakes

Beginning students make some errors in the initial interview that are common enough to mention at this point. Students either become too task oriented or too person oriented. That is, they become overly concerned with gathering information and neglect the client's concerns; or they are overly concerned with the client's feelings and, as a result, end up with little or no information. A balance between the two extremes is the goal you should work toward.

Another, related error is that of providing too little structure and directiveness, letting the client totally guide the topics to be discussed. It is not uncommon for the client to overwhelm the interviewer with words. Students who are learning therapy often find it relatively easy to fulfill the role of accepting and supportive listener, yet find it much more difficult to provide the structure required for a productive interview.

Beginners also often have difficulty in assessing whether they have pursued an area in enough detail. They often ask a general question or two about a problem area and find that the client's contributions stop. Not wanting to push the client too much, they then skip to another problem area and proceed with another superficial coverage of these issues. As a result of experience in interviewing, students will come to realize when they have sufficient understanding of a situation or a problem; however, at first, they generally tend to have insufficient information.

A similar mistake beginners make is that of assuming that they understand what the client is saying without carefully checking out their assumptions. We remind students to assume nothing, to question their clients closely to ascertain exactly what they mean. Although both students and clients may think they are dealing with obvious matters, it is surprising how often misunderstandings occur. For example:

> A tense man entered therapy because of vaguely stated difficulties he was having in communicating with his boss and in controlling his temper at work. On occasion he made reference to "losing it," which the interviewer assumed meant losing his temper. On closer questioning during the next interview, the client revealed fears about losing control and "going crazy," which added a totally new dimension to the clinical picture he was presenting.

Unless the therapist asks about the client's exact meaning, some form of serious misunderstanding may occur. Students and clients may think that they *both* know what it means to feel anxious, down, uncertain, helpless, inadequate, and so on. However, what the client means when using these words to describe his or her experience and what the therapist understands may be very dissimilar. Misunderstanding may result from confusion about *degree* or *amount* of a feeling or about the behaviors involved. For example, *down* may mean feeling tired and unhappy to the therapist, but it may mean the inability to leave the house and suicidal thoughts to the client.

Private aspects of people's lives, such as sex and finances, may be clinically very important but are often superficially covered by beginners. Clients find these difficult to discuss, and student therapists often find it inordinately difficult to question people about these matters.

42

In their concern not to offend a client by exploring "taboo" areas or intruding, students may implicitly communicate that discussion of such topics is not acceptable. The therapist's discomfort about "prying" may mask a personal concern about discussing private matters with any but family or intimate friends. Therapists are not automatically equipped to be able to discuss such topics as sex, rage, hallucinations, suicide, and homosexuality. It requires concerted effort and practice to be comfortable in dealing with such areas and to communicate this comfort to clients, but this is an essential part of the learning process. You model in this area by being direct and forthright yet accepting and understanding of the uneasiness involved.

Because the initial interview is the client's first contact with the therapist, it is an extremely important event. Creating an accepting climate and giving the client the opportunity to begin to clarify his or her problems are your general goals. A successful first interview is an important base from which to build your subsequent treatment relationship.

5

Consultations

The assessment stage of therapy frequently involves consultations with other agencies or professionals involved with your client. Securing relevant information from others about a client and using the information judiciously and fairly is a skill requiring considerable experience and clinical judgment. In this chapter we discuss the reasons for obtaining information from sources other than the client, the types of information to be obtained, and how to approach the client and the consultant about your request. In addition, we deal with the more difficult judgmental task of using the information once it has been acquired.

There are a variety of reasons for consulting with other sources of information about your client. It can be extremely helpful in your treatment planning to speak to a client's previous therapist concerning his or her impressions of the client, the goals and progress of therapy, and the reason for termination. Moreover, the ethics of most professions dictate that you be given as much information as possible about your client. Other professional opinions are considered to be uniquely informative and must be obtained and evaluated. In addition, you may be liable for malpractice if something unforeseen happens to the client during treatment and you have not made a consultation that might have provided relevant information.

Whom to ask for information

Previous therapists. An obvious source of information concerning a new client is a client's previous therapist. Perhaps the most useful information you will obtain is the attitude the client displayed toward therapy and the difficulties the therapist encountered. For example:

> A young male client who appeared to be confused, anxious, and disorganized reported that his previous therapist had terminated treatment with him. Consultation with that therapist revealed that the patient had been unreliable about making and keeping appointments, had been difficult to keep focused on the business of therapy, and had left therapy without informing the therapist.

In this case the consultation allowed the new therapist to anticipate problems that did in fact occur with this client. He was able to eliminate some of the difficulties by making a firm contract with the client that clearly spelled out the conditions for treatment (e.g., making and keeping appointments on time and paying at each session).

Another example:

> A woman brought her seven-year-old daughter to therapy because of problems with obedience at school, inability to make friends, and difficulty concentrating. The child's previous therapist reported that he perceived the major problem to be the mother's difficulty in managing her child. Furthermore, he believed that the mother was resistant to becoming involved in therapy and had terminated treatment when pressure was put on her to attend sessions.

The new therapist's awareness of the mother's possible reluctance to become involved resulted in her focusing immediately on this issue before any other treatment occurred. Although the mother's resistance was never entirely resolved, she did agree to participate in family treatment and ultimately came to see her role in the problem.

A third example:

> A client told her new therapist that she had terminated her previous therapy because she was making no progress toward solving her problems of fearfulness and obsessive thinking. The client's previous therapist was an older woman who assumed a motherly, supportive role with the client. She commented that the client's fears of dependency resulted in anxiety about the helping situation and subsequent flight from it.

As a result of this information the new therapist chose to take a less supportive and directive stance with the client. This maximized her feelings of independence and comfort within the therapy situation and prevented another premature termination.

In the preceding examples the information gained through consultation was crucial to the treatment planning. It is quite helpful to be able to anticipate the client's possible reactions to you and to therapy on the basis of his or her actual behavioral response to a similar past situation. Of course, the client may have changed, the current situation may be different from the past one, or the therapist may have misperceived the events reported. However, more often than not we've found that predictions based on past behavior in therapy have been accurate. Most importantly, these predictions have allowed the therapist to plan treatment so as to maximize the chances for success.

Consulting with previous treatment providers may also help resolve difficult questions about diagnosis and treatment. The former therapist may have seen the client at a time when the nature of the problems was more obvious. For example:

> A client requested therapy for confusion and depression of unknown origin. Consultation with a previous therapist revealed that the client had been hospitalized for a psychotic episode following the death of her father.

This information alerted the therapist to the possibility of the client's decompensating and made him look carefully for signs of difficulty and disorganization in her daily functioning. As a consequence, another hospitalization was avoided by frequent supportive therapy sessions.

Contacting previous therapists may be useful in a variety of other situations: for example, in confirming or adding new (or omitted) information to what has been provided by the client; in resolving contradictions in what the client has said; and in alerting you to the possibility of manipulation or impulsive behavior. Obtaining another perspective on the client and his or her problems can in itself be quite helpful. A previous therapist who has seen the client for any length of time will probably know him or her better, or at least in different ways, than will an intake interviewer who has seen the client only once or twice.

It seems appropriate at this point to raise the issue of the special problems that arise when a client who requests therapy from you has not yet terminated with another therapist. You should be cautious about making a therapy contract with an individual in this situation. The ethics of professional practice dictate that you avoid undermining the treatment efforts of another therapist. In addition to the ethical issue, however, there is also a treatment issue involved. Clients may leave treatment out of reluctance to deal with the issues being raised. Someone who comes to you asking for help may have unfinished business that may best be resolved with the previous therapist. In the interests of the client's treatment it is wise to encourage him or her to return to the therapist and discuss the desire to terminate.

Health practitioners. A psychotherapist is ethically required to consult with any person currently providing help in order to gain information relevant to the treatment, to ascertain whether the two treatments are compatible, and to inform the other professional of the proposed treatment plan. This is particularly important with ongoing psychiatric or medical treatment, where non-medical therapists may be liable for suit if something happens to the client and relevant consultations have not been made. Consulting with the other professionals involved has the added advantage of ensuring that the client will not receive confusing or incompatible suggestions and that he or she will not be able to use one professional's suggestion to discredit the other.

Following are some examples of cases where consultation with a physician was made that proved to be valuable to the nonmedical psychotherapist's treatment:

A young woman requested therapy for depression, fatigue, binge eating, and difficulty sleeping. In addition, she mentioned that her physician had diagnosed her as hypoglycemic. Knowing that hypoglycemia often results in symptoms similar to depression, the therapist requested a consultation. The physician reported that the patient herself had brought up the issue of physical illness and that he had merely mentioned the possibility of hypoglycemia. Further blood sugar tests did not confirm the diagnosis. As a consequence, the therapist was more secure about pursuing the psychological causes of the patient's symptoms in therapy.

An obese thirty-year-old male bookkeeper requested therapy for a severe depression, which had resulted in his having to quit his job. His current family physician was consulted; he reported that the client was taking a total of seven medications, including ones for sleep, severe back pain, hypertension, and anxiety. In this case the new therapist requested a complete medication reevaluation from a physician trained in the use and complications of psychoactive drugs. Only then could he adequately evaluate the psychological status of the client.

Schools. When children under eighteen are brought to therapy it is essential to consult with the teacher, counselor, and principal of the child's school. The school day is a large part of the child's life, and it is quite possible that any problems the child has at home may affect his or her school performance. In addition, the school personnel will often provide additional information and another perspective on the difficulties.

The following example demonstrates a case in which consultation with the school provided information crucial to effective treatment:

> A mother brought her eight-year-old boy to a therapist because she had been told by school personnel that her child was gifted. She wanted an assessment of his intelligence as well as recommendations for school placement. On consultation with the child's teacher, the therapist learned that the mother had apparently misunderstood a remark made at a parent conference and, moreover, that the child was not functioning up to the average level of the class, even though he gave some evidence of being quite bright.

In addition to the value of the teacher's observations of the child's problems, schools often have very valuable testing and previous treatment records that may save you and the client a good deal of time and redundant effort. For example:

> A young boy was brought to the clinic because his parents feared he was a slow learner and was somehow different from the other children. Prior test reports obtained from the school indicated a decrease of abilities during the past two years. The severity of the drop in functioning indicated the possibility of a progressive brain tumor.

In addition to collecting useful information, consultation with a child's school at an early point in treatment will avoid misunderstandings and duplication of effort. The treatment of a school-age child frequently involves school personnel and may require considerable cooperation and effort on their part. The school is a large, significant portion of the child's environment, and lack of cooperation there may completely sabotage your treatment efforts. Your chances of success in implementing a coordinated treatment plan will be increased by considering the school personnel's information about the child's problem and their point of view regarding the potential and limits of the classroom as a treatment setting.

Other possible consultations. We've mentioned in some detail the more frequently encountered situations in which information from other sources is relevant to making an assessment of the client's problems. Psychological consultations, in which psychological tests are used to evaluate a client, can provide a valuable second opinion to the therapist. A variety of psychological assessment techniques are useful additions to the interview. Some of the more commonly used measures are personality questionnaires; projective tests; intelligence, special ability, and disability tests; and tests to determine neurological damage.

Another possible source of information is the agency or professional who referred the client for therapy. In addition, some clients will have had contact with a social service agency, with the courts, or with correction facilities. Information from these contacts may significantly affect your assessment of the client's problems and his or her current situation.

How to approach the client

You may not reveal anything about a client, even his or her name, without written permission. Requesting that a client sign a release of information form to allow you to consult with a previous treatment provider is often a delicate and complicated situation. Although you may believe that the information is important, you do not want to damage your relationship with the client by aggravating concerns about confidentiality. This is a distinct possiblity, particularly at the early stages of therapy.

You must remember that it is the client's right to refuse to allow you to speak with anyone else about him or her. Some clients will sign away their privilege with very little concern. Others, however, will want to know exactly what you intend to ask the consultant, what you plan to tell him or her, and will demand a full report of the information you received. It is important to clarify with the client what the consultation will and will not involve before making any outside contact. Coming to an agreement before you seek the information will avoid misunderstandings or hard feelings later.

We make it a practice to tell the informational source as little about the client as possible, even though the release of information is for a "mutual exchange." It's a good idea to discuss with the client in some depth his or her feelings about the outside contact in order to determine what might be best left unsaid. Our guidelines are to tell the individual only that the client is seeking treatment at our clinic, but we usually avoid discussing the nature of the problem, our initial impressions, or the client's current situation unless it is necessary.

Of course, in some instances more specificity is called for, such as in a consultation with a gynecologist when a woman is seeking sexual therapy. The physician would be unable to make the appropriate examination without knowing the nature of the problem. Also, if the other professional has ongoing treatment responsibility for the client, you will probably need to provide more comprehensive information. All these issues should be clarified fully between you and the client before seeking out the information.

When the client refuses to sign a release of information you must be prepared to evaluate how critical that piece of information is to your treatment and what the ethical and legal implications are in continuing therapy without it. When the therapist feels that the client's refusal will create serious practical, ethical, or legal obstacles to treatment, he or she may not be willing to make a contract with the client. For example:

> Parents requested therapy for their daughter at the recommendation of the juvenile court. The girl had been arrested for possession of alcohol, and her participation in family therapy was a condition for parole. Although the

51

family had been in therapy previously, the mother refused to sign a release for the new therapist to consult with the previous one. She claimed that the prior treatment had been ineffective and that her confidence in the current therapy would be undermined if it were prejudiced by the prior therapist's impressions.

In this situation the new therapist refused to continue the treatment assessment without having access to the previous therapist's information, believing that he could not make an adequate assessment of the family for treatment while lacking this resource.

Another example:

A suspicious, sensitive young woman requested therapy for difficulties she was having in communicating with people that resulted in losing her friends. She told the therapist about having been seen previously at the student counseling center, where she had felt acutely uncomfortable. When asked for her signature allowing that consultation, she refused, commenting that she had already told the new therapist everything she had told the previous one and more.

In this case the therapist chose to honor the feelings of the client in the interests of maintaining a relationship with her. He feared that the client would have left therapy immediately if he had pushed her on this issue, and the therapist felt that involving this client in an effective therapeutic relationship was crucial for her stability.

How to approach the consultant

The person from whom you are seeking information must have the signed release form in hand before being able legally to give you any information. Our cover letter accompanying the copy of the signed release form identifies the client and the therapist and mentions that the therapist will be following up the letter with a telephone call. It's usually best to call the consultant rather than wait for a report, since you may have to wait a long time for a written reply.

We recommend that students identify themselves, their organization, and the client on the telephone and have a prepared list of questions to ask. Frequently the therapist and supervisor discuss areas in which information is desired. The questions are determined by the type of contact, the nature of our needs for information, and the confidentiality concerns of the client. If you provide some structure regarding what you want to know, the consultant will be able to focus more clearly on relevant issues and will be more useful to you.

You will no doubt encounter some individuals who will refuse to give you any information at all, even with the client's consent. You will also probably encounter therapists who keep no written records. By and large, however, you will usually find that colleagues you contact will be eager to be helpful.

During your discussion with the consultant you should clarify what you will be telling the client about the information you receive. An understood standard of professional practice is that information received through a consultation of this sort is given for the specific purpose of assisting the new therapist in his or her treatment efforts. It is not assumed that such information is revealed to the client in any detail. If you intend to disclose the information to the client in any but a general way, you must inform your contact of that fact. Although the other professional does not have the same legal confidentiality privilege as that afforded to the client, you are ethically bound to tell him or her how you intend to use the information.

How to use the information obtained from a consultation

One of the more difficult tasks for the beginning therapist is deciding how to use the information received from consultations, particularly when it is contradictory to your own impressions or what the client has told you. It is important to keep an open mind about the contradictions and carefully consider the implications of the differing impressions or facts. Beginners tend to rush into action, confronting the client prematurely about a possible misrepresentation or distortion. For example:

> A young married couple with two children requested sex therapy to deal with problems of painful intercourse. Their difficulties had recently been exacerbated by the wife's contracting gonorrhea from an extramarital affair and infecting the husband. The therapist suspected that the wife was interested in dissolving the marriage but was unable to confront her husband with her lack of commitment. An outside consultation with her gynecologist revealed that the client had had several previous affairs, which she denied to the therapist.

Although the therapist wanted to ask her about the contradiction, he decided to wait until it seemed necessary. Contrary to his expectations, the therapy proceeded smoothly, and he was no longer concerned about her commitment to the marriage.

Student therapists tend to discredit information from professionals from a different theoretical school or discipline. They also dismiss impressions that differ from their own or from the client's representation of himself or herself. This is shortsightedness on the part of the beginner. Even though the information is couched in terms you may dislike or not understand, don't dismiss it. You may find the additional perspective to be useful in conceptualizing treatment, or you may later discover that your initial impressions were in error. Beginners tend to be threatened by contradictory information, as if their own impressions are suspect or worthless because of it. The key to dealing with this situation is to consider all the aspects of the disagreement carefully with your supervisor before you make a judgment or decide on a course of action.

Students also believe that in order to be "honest" they must report the full content of the information they receive from the consultant to the client. Actually, it is your ethical responsibility not to share the information indiscriminately. As mentioned previously, this is a violation of professional ethics. It is difficult to determine how much information to share with a client, and the decision should be given considerable thought. Generally we suggest that the therapist translate the information into general comments. What you reveal will depend very much on what you and your supervisor think will be helpful to your therapy, and what you actually decide in each case will vary tremendously from client to client.

Ongoing consultation during treatment

Although consultations during the assessment phase of therapy may provide very useful information for treatment choice and planning, they may also set the stage for ongoing contact during the course of therapy. You may wish to keep regular contact with a physician, for example, who is supervising the client's medications. Regular contact will allow you to evaluate the possible effects of the medication on the patient's psychological state and to request changes if the medication is not having the desired effect.

Such give and take will minimize the possibility of the client's being confused by differing professional opinions or taking advantage of differences to avoid making changes. You will increase your effectiveness in therapy tremendously if you consider and use the other resources in the client's environment to reinforce further the changes made in therapy.

6

Giving a staffing report

The preceding chapters have attempted to provide you with a step-by-step framework for making an assessment of your client for psychotherapy. At this point we hope to provide some structure and assistance for the final and possibly most important ingredient in the assessment process, the staffing (intake) report. Many clinical training and treatment settings utilize a conference format at which the interviewer presents a formal report on the intake process to the clinic staff and trainees. This report typically consists of an oral presentation of the interviewer's assessment of the client as derived from interviews and other available information.

The ability to communicate a clinical picture of your client to a group of colleagues is critical in making such a presentation. You must evaluate all the information you have about the client and present it in an organized, concise, and clear manner. Although this is often a time-consuming and difficult task for the student, it is the heart of the initial evaluation process. The formulation of a staffing report is of unequaled value as a training exercise because it requires you to weigh all the information you have gathered and draw on all the skills you have learned.

The staffing conference serves other purposes as well within clinical settings. The training staff uses the conference format as a way of monitoring students' skills in conceptualizing cases. In addition, it is an ideal setting for exposing trainees to a variety of clinical problems and different theoretical perspectives. The presentation of case material is useful for generating discussion of disposition, treatment, and diagnostic issues that will add to your clinical knowledge and increase your experience.

The report format also provides the opportunity for staff members to communicate their information and conclusions regarding clients to a group of other clinicians. It exposes the intake interviewer to additional opinions about the client and potential treatment approaches. The discussion generated by the presenter's ideas can be very lively. Staff members will often disagree vigorously in their opinions about a client. The consensus reached after such a discussion will incorporate the ideas of diverse clinicians with different experiences and orientations. Besides serving a crucial training function, then, it also gives the client the advantage of having many clinicians consider and evaluate his or her problems and make recommendations for treatment.

We've discussed the importance of the staffing conference in terms of how it functions within a training setting. However, from the beginner's point of view, it is possibly the most threatening of all the demands in clinical training. You have just started to see clients, which itself causes anxiety. You are unsure of your ability to gather information, you don't trust your own judgments, and you are asked to present your ideas to a group of your colleagues for their critical review and feedback.

The staffing report involves difficult factual and judgmental decisions that you will not be prepared to handle completely in the first stages of your training. Your supervisors and fellow staff members expect that their comments will be helpful, not threatening, to you. Taken in this way, the staffing conference can be an invaluable training tool.

In this chapter we will present a frame of reference for you to use in preparing your report. We will also attempt to direct our comments to the common questions generated by worried students: What do I say? How do I say it?

57

What if someone disagrees with me? What if I forget to include an important fact? Although we cannot eliminate all the anxieties inherent in the situation and the fears of oral presentation, we hope that our framework will provide some relief and support in coping with the task and will assist you in making a more effective presentation.

Organizing the information

The key to giving a good staffing report with a minimum of discomfort is thorough preparation. You will be attempting to communicate a considerable amount of information to your audience; talking "off the top of your head" in this situation never works. It is crucial to have a well-organized plan and to know your information well. The plan should include the relevant information presented succinctly in a logical, step-by-step sequence. We will describe one general model for organizing your staffing report that can be altered to fit the requirements of your setting and clientele. There are other models currently in use in clinical practice that will also provide an adequate frame of reference. What is important is that you use some method of structuring how you think through your information and draw conclusions. We will first discuss our model as a guide for organizing your thinking and later consider the skills involved in the actual oral presentation.

Orienting information. To begin with, it is useful to imagine that your listeners know nothing whatsoever about the case you are going to present. In order for them to understand the facts and issues and to be able to visualize the client, you will need to present some orienting information. By this we mean pertinent facts about the client that identify him or her with regard to sex, age, occupation, marital status, living situation, and referral source. In fact, you will probably find your listeners later interrupting your report to ask for this specific identifying information if you neglect to provide it initially. It is also quite useful to include some descriptive comments about the outstanding or clinically relevant physical character-istics, mannerisms, or interpersonal style of the client. This will provide a framework for your listeners within which to place the information that follows:

> The client is an obese, single, thirty-five-year-old unem-ployed woman who lives with her widowed father. She was referred to therapy by her family physician, who was concerned about the effect of her weight on her health.

> The client is a short, slight, fourteen-year-old male high school sophomore who was brought to therapy by his father and stepmother at the suggestion of his school counselor.

Including short selections from your interviews with audio or video tape can be a very useful adjunct to the descriptive material that you present at the start of the report. The use of a carefully edited piece of tape can communicate the "flavor" of a client very effectively – his or her style of speaking and relating, mood, posture, tone of voice, and any unusual mannerisms or characteristics.

Presenting problem. The brief orienting information is usually followed by a direct statement of the problem as the client describes it. The term *presenting problem* re-fers to the client's stated reason for wanting therapy. It is the cornerstone from which the entire report is devel-oped. You should try to represent as accurately as possi-ble how the client reports his or her difficulties, even though you may not agree that this is in fact your client's major problem. This section of the report calls for stating what the client said without embellishing or interpreting it, a mistake students often make. For example:

> A thirty-year-old woman applied for therapy, stating that she wanted help for her compulsive overeating. Her hus-band had left her and their two children only three days previously, and she believed that her weight was the cause of their separation.

59

Even though this client was obviously greatly distressed about the breakup of her marriage, she chose to select her weight as the problem to present for therapy. Therefore the individual making the staffing presentation should accurately reflect her initial focus and perspective.

In the presenting problem section you should also discuss the onset and course of the presenting problem: when it was first noticed, its changes over time, and its effects on the client's life. It is customary to include a description of the client's feelings and behaviors associated with the problem, the situations in which it occurs, and the short- and long-term consequences. Some individuals will have made attempts to solve the problem before coming to you for help, and mention should be made of these efforts and the results. Finally, try to address the following questions: Why is the client seeking help now? What events led up to the application for therapy at this time? The following is an example of a presenting problem section:

> The client, a college sophomore, is seeking therapy because of her inability to receive hypodermic injections without fainting. She reports feeling humiliated by the problem and fearful of being embarrassed in public. Even anticipating receiving a shot results in severe anxiety and nausea.
>
> She remembers fainting for the first time at age seven, after receiving a shot from her dentist. She has had the same reaction to injections ever since. In addition, the client often feels faint when viewing others receiving shots in movies or on television. This is usually accompanied by slight nausea and light-headedness.
>
> For the past few years the client has avoided any situations that involve the possibility of her receiving a hypodermic injection. She has applied for help with this problem now because she has been accepted to an overseas campus and must receive some inoculations in order to secure a passport.

From the student's point of view, it is not always easy to distill what the client believes to be the problem and its ramifications from the mass of interview material. The problems themselves will range in specificity from vague discomfort to an elaborate analysis of intrapsychic conflicts. Your task at this point in the presentation is to convey to your listeners as clearly as possible the client's concerns at the level of specificity and depth that the client presented them to you.

Current functioning. The presenting problem section is followed by a description of the client's current functioning. The term *current functioning* refers to a discussion of the client's present situation and an evaluation of how he or she is coping with a broad range of life issues. It usually includes a cross-section view of the individual's living circumstances, marital situation, social life, health, finances, occupation, religion, and leisure activities. Any other aspects relevant to the presenting problem should be discussed. An abbreviated example follows:

> The client is currently unemployed and has been for the last six months. He recently ran out of unemployment benefits and was forced to move back home with his mother and father. He has no occupational or career interests and does not know what kind of job he wants. He spends most of his time alone at home or engaged in solitary activities, such as jogging. He reports avoiding his friends to the point of not even answering the phone when it rings. He does not date and reports having no sexual feelings. He derives enjoyment from none of his activities, with the exception of drinking alcohol.

Commonly you will give relatively greater emphasis to those areas that appear to affect or to be affected by the client's presenting problem. For example, an adolescent girl suffering from tics may also experience repercussions in her social life. This might warrant some extended discussion in your report. On the other hand, if your client is an aging businessman troubled by insomnia and heart attacks, you might want to discuss his occupational life and current health in more detail. In any event, you should be sure to convey to your listeners some general idea of the client's overall level of functioning by surveying, at least briefly, all areas.

Supporting history. Inclusion of historical material at this point in your report serves a very important function. It provides support and further evidence on which to base your speculations, impressions, and proposed treatment plan. In addition, selected aspects of the client's history may reveal patterns that will give consistency to your picture of the client's ways of behaving and support for your diagnostic impressions and prognosis. Remember that you are trying to convey a broad understanding of the client through the details of his or her life history.

You may find that you have gathered more historical information than is necessary or possible to convey in your report. This problem is only resolved with increased experience, which allows you to judge the most significant areas to pursue. If they have sufficient interviewing time, students tend to question broadly and thoroughly in all historical areas – family, social, medical, educational, marital, and occupational. It is particularly critical in this section of the report that you select relevant information carefully.

Unfortunately, we cannot spell out in detail how to go about selecting and organizing the historical information to include in each report. As with all other aspects of clinical practice, each client will dictate a slightly different approach. However, we can give you some general guidelines. An intake report usually includes some mention of the client's early family life and the quality of the family interactions. It also conveys information concerning his or her school, social, and occupational development and adjustment over the years. Any unusual, erratic, or atypical events should be noted, as should any significant medical information or illnesses. It is often helpful to the listener if you provide brief summary statements for areas not of vital importance – for example,

"The client's work history is unremarkable," or, "He was inexperienced sexually until his marriage."

Listening to a detailed account of the job history of a particular client, for example, may bore your listeners to inattention. On the other hand, this same information may be crucial to understanding another client's problem. There is a wealth of information to be gathered during an interview. The difficult part, as we have said, lies in the careful selection and reporting of only the information that adds to your listeners' understanding of the client.

Testing and consultations. Once you have related what you have been told by the client, you should turn your attention to sources of information other than the interview. Primary among those sources are consultations with other professionals or agencies and testing results. This information may be extremely useful in formulating a picture of the client and deriving the most appropriate treatment plan.

Although you have had relatively brief exposure to the client, you may have access to greater information about the client's behavior from his or her contact with other people. An in-depth discussion of consultations occurs in Chapter 5. However, we want to emphasize here that including the information gathered through consultations may be exceptionally valuable to the staffing procedure, particularly if the source is a previous therapist. From the intake interviews you have only the client's report and your own judgmental inference from which to draw conclusions; however, consultation with another therapist may tell you considerably more about the client's ways of solving problems and about how he or she used therapy in the past. It also provides some measure of the client's objectivity about his or her problems. This type of information may be the deciding factor in choosing a particular treatment approach and may prevent another therapeutic failure.

Likewise, material derived from testing may be a significant part of the staffing report, depending on the nature of test data available to you. For example, if the client is a child whose problem involves school behavior, summarizing the results of a battery including intelligence and achievement tests will be critical to the assessment of the problem and to an appropriate treatment plan. Although this may be a particularly obvious example, it is only one of the many situations where testing provides critical input to a staffing report.

In summary, it is to your advantage to include information from a variety of sources in your report. You and your listeners will be more confident of your conclusions when such additional relevant information is brought to bear on the decision-making process.

Clinical judgments. Up to this point your report has consisted basically of a collection of facts about the client. Although students have some difficulty with the previous sections, they tend to have the most difficulty with the remaining parts of the report – those that call for making inferences and drawing conclusions about the client. It is important to keep in mind that all the other information has been offered to provide a context for the judgments and recommendations you are now asked to make. These are essentially the heart of the report.

In making clinical judgments you are required to assess all the previously presented information about the client from a different framework. That framework is your knowledge and clinical experience regarding normal and problematic behavior. Since as beginners your experience will be limited, you will probably have difficulty in designating the parameters of unusual, peculiar, or disturbed behavior. Students find that they often need to draw on the experience of their supervisors to make such decisions.

Clinical impressions are your opinions about the client and the nature of his or her problems, based on your academic knowledge, practical training, and experience.

They usually involve judgments about the client's personality structure, motivations, needs, and conflicts. There are some acknowledged dimensions that are usually included in these judgments. These may include (1) the client's current emotional state or mood; (2) his or her ability to think and to recall information clearly; (3) his or her ability to perceive external reality without distortion; (4) his or her level of subjective discomfort; and (5) some general statement regarding the client's level of disturbance or inability to function. The aim of these statements, sometimes called the client's *mental status*, is to identify unusual or pathological qualities in the client's interview behavior, thinking, perceptions, and affect. Following are three examples of clinical judgments that may help to clarify this task for you:

The client is highly anxious, agitated, and restless. He reacts to emotionally charged material with intensity. His thinking is disorganized, and he has difficulty stating things in a concrete or specific manner. He is unable to recall events from his past, but his ability to perceive reality in the present seems intact. He is severely disturbed but still able to respond appropriately to a structured interview situation. When in a less structured situation, he becomes considerably more disorganized, irrelevant, and incoherent.

The client tries very hard to appear unemotional and in complete control of himself and the situation. He appears to be of above-average intelligence and is logical in his thinking. However, he can be very vague in relating events about which he is reluctant to talk. The client's memory is clear and detailed, with the exception of recall of the emotional content of his experiences. He appears to be in good contact with reality and demonstrates no evidence of any unusual experiences.

Although the client reported problems with depression, she did not appear to be depressed at either interview, but was tense and animated. She seems to be of average intelligence, although her thinking reveals an illogical quality. Rather than evidence of pathology, this lack of logic seems to be due to careless, adolescent thinking. She had some difficulty remembering dates and the order of events, though this again seems to be within the normal range and mainly the result of unorganized thinking. Her perceptual processes are undisturbed.

Note regarding diagnoses. Your clinical judgments, as previously described, form the basis for a *diagnostic formulation.* This term refers to a summary discussion of the nature and severity of the client's disorder. Many clinical settings will require you to formulate your ideas in the specific form of a diagnostic category selected from the *Diagnostic and Statistical Manual* (DSM II); others will not. However, some statement of a diagnostic formulation is a necessary ingredient in your presentation and sets the stage for discussing appropriate treatment recommendations. In deciding whether to use a standard diagnosis to describe your client you should consider whether the label will accurately represent the nature of the difficulty and will bring some additional knowledge to bear on your understanding of the client's problems. For example, the categories of depression and psychosis, when appropriate, are critical to your listeners' understanding of the client. On the other hand, if your client is complaining of orgasmic dysfunction, the appropriate label, "psychophysiologic genitourinary disorder," carries little explanatory value.

Treatment recommendations. The final part of the staffing presentation is a proposal regarding the appropriate treatment plan for this particular person with this particular set of problems. Ideally, the student will consider all the foregoing information together with his or her knowledge of treatment methodologies to formulate a set of goals for the client and the appropriate method for reaching them.

The first issue to be addressed is the disposition of the case. Basically, is some form of psychotherapeutic treatment appropriate for the client, and should the person be accepted for treatment in your setting? If you think that the client should be offered treatment, and if your setting offers appropriate services, you should present a clear and specific set of goals for treatment. In some instances the client will specify certain goals he or she has for coming to therapy. You will want to discuss the client's goals together with your own perceptions of his or her problems. There will be cases in which your treatment goals do not precisely coincide with the client's, and the differences should be explored thoroughly in your report. Dealing with these differences with the client is a complicated clinical task and will be discussed thoroughly in the next chapter.

After specifying the goals of therapy you should describe the type of treatment method you propose to use in reaching these goals. The treatment methodology should have a clear conceptual and practical relationship to the proposed changes to be made by the client. Besides discussing how you propose to work with the client, you should discuss why you selected this approach as opposed to other alternatives. In addition, any special considerations relevant to the treatment of the client should be mentioned: for example, preference for sex of therapist, use of medications as an adjunct to therapy, and concerns about suicide or hospitalization. You may also want to mention any particular difficulties you anticipate in working with the client and how you plan to deal with them. In addition, the risks of proceeding or not proceeding with treatment should be discussed and evaluated.

Finally, you should conclude your recommendations with a statement about the prognosis, or your opinion of the client's chances of successful treatment. This statement includes a consideration of the client's apparent motivation to change, the environmental factors that will enhance or obstruct the work of therapy, and the nature of the problems themselves and their duration.

The following is an example of treatment recommendations for a young woman who presented problems with excessive drinking:

> The goals of treatment are as follows: (1) to decrease the amount of alcohol consumed and established new patterns of drinking; and (2) to help the client develop alternative ways of coping with stress and depression. A behaviorally oriented self-control program for drinking is recommended. This program would involve identifying the situations that resulted in the client's drinking, developing alternative responses in these situations, and implementing a contingency system to maintain the desired behaviors. It appears that the client will function best in a fairly structured environment with minimal stress; if she learns to restructure her work and social environment along these lines, her chances of maintaining a lower drinking level are fairly good.

Another example:

> Major goals of treatment are to help the client gain control over his tension and obsessive sexual fears and to provide him with appropriate social skills. A cautious, supportive approach is recommended for the initial phase of treatment, along with continued evaluation of his level of awareness and ability to handle discussion of his sexual identity. The focus of therapy will be on current stressful events and on developing more appropriate ways of dealing with his feelings, particularly anger. Helping the client recognize his strengths and gain confidence will hopefully weaken his passive, helpless view of himself and facilitate more active coping strategies.

Making a staffing presentation

In this chapter we have offered a framework for organizing your thoughts about a client prior to giving an oral staffing presentation. Giving the actual report involves some additional skills; these include a verbal presentation that is clear, concise, and organized.

Communicating clinical material. Few students are naturally able to communicate information and impressions about a client in an effective manner. It is a difficult task, requiring extensive preparation and repeated practice. As an intake interviewer you will be faced with the task of sorting the relevant and significant from an overwhelming mass of data about a client. It is tempting to include everything you have learned about the client and his or her situation in the report for fear of leaving out something important. This indiscriminate approach to report presentation leaves your listeners with the impossible task of sorting through all the detail to discern the crucial points. This is quite distracting to the listener, who is attempting to grasp the critical information quickly and, simultaneously, to formulate his or her own opinions.

We can provide some general guidelines on communicating clinical material in a staffing report. It is of critical importance to be clear and concise and not to use language you do not fully understand or cannot define. Having your report organized in a thoughtful and logical manner is also essential in getting your points across. Many students make the mistake of presenting the information as the client presented it in the interviews. In order to be readily understandable to the other listeners, you will need to impose a structure on what the client says. It is also critically important to weigh the material that you have gathered in terms of its relevance to the purposes of the report. Not all pieces of information have equal priority in this regard. What you choose to include should reflect your conceptualization of the situation and should help to clarify your reasoning for your listeners.

Being thorough enough without being overly detailed or redundant is quite difficult, particularly in your first reports. With experience you will begin to be able to make those discriminations yourself. Paying attention to the questions that members of the supervisory staff ask you at the presentation will alert you to clinically significant pieces of information that you will want to include the next time.

69

Two examples here may be helpful. The first is an initial statement that is cluttered by irrelevant detail; the second, on the same client, is concise and to the point:

> The client came to the clinic on the referral of the doctor whom he was seeing for a skin problem. The doctor felt that we could be of service to this young man, who experiences considerably anxiety when taking tests, particularly in the sciences. The client was ten minutes late for his interview and explained that he had trouble finding parking near the clinic.

> The client is a twenty-three-year-old single male who is seeking help for test anxiety; he was referred for therapy by the student health center. He is currently enrolled in the university as a sophomore and is under considerable pressure to maintain a grade-point average of 2.0 in order to keep his scholarship.

Your goal should be to offer the information in a straightforward way so that your listeners can draw their own conclusions. Language that is either too casual or too formal will detract from your presentation. Again, students often err in both directions. Some present their material in an obscure and intellectualized fashion; others try to be folksy or to capture the flavor of the client's style of talking. Your listeners will be much more impressed by (and, incidentally, grateful for) a clear and easily understood presentation than by a labored or complex one.

Handling your anxieties about oral reports. Sharing your responsibility for decision making about the client with your audience at the staffing conference theoretically should make you more comfortable about practicing clinical work while you are in training. Reaching a consensus within a group of clinicians brings more expertise to bear on the ethical issues and practical decisions involved in treatment planning. As a consequence, you can be more confident in the appropriateness of the resulting plan and of your ability to treat the client competently.

However, students often find that their anxiety about

evaluation in these situations is very great. They tend to become preoccupied with not being wrong. This concern may lead to defending their impressions and treatment plan rather than to listening to other people's suggestions and ideas. Don't feel the need to respond or to have an answer to every comment, criticism, or alternative hypothesis. This defeats the major purpose of the conference. It is a great strength in this situation to be able and willing to discuss, consider, and evaluate feedback, alternatives, and opinions.

Clearly, this is a difficult thing to ask. Students have invested a great deal of time and effort in preparing these reports, and their own feelings of self-esteem and competence mistakenly rest on their ability to generate agreement with their perceptions. It is threatening to have missed an interpretation or to have disregarded an important piece of information. Moreover, many students are afraid of looking bad in front of their supervisors and peers and expect that they should have found the "right" answer themselves.

Actually, it is impossible to predict what consensus will be generated out of a group of clinicians with different perspectives and different interests. It is a matter of judgment rather than of right versus wrong. To expend a great deal of energy attempting to please everyone is self-defeating. You then invest so much in your answer that you cannot benefit from the opinions of others.

This seems to be a universal problem for students, who have been brought up in the competitive and evaluation-oriented world of academic training. As we've mentioned earlier, the ability to admit you are mistaken and to be able to listen to feedback and to learn from people whose opinions differ from yours is crucial to the psychotherapy training process. Making a staffing presentation can be one of the more anxiety-provoking aspects of your training. However, when it is approached with the spirit of sharing knowledge and experience, it can also be one of the most profitable.

Part III

The psychotherapy process

7
Beginning therapy: feedback and contracting

A key point in the evaluation and treatment process arrives when the interviewer relates back to the client his or her professional judgments and presents recommendations for treatment. This feedback interview is a most important time for clients. They have related their concerns to you and have tried to respond to the range of questions you have asked. Now they wait eagerly for your opinions about these problems and for your decisions about treatment. This is also an important time for the interviewer. You know that your client will give each word considerable weight and that his or her decision about treatment and later progress will in part depend on the effectiveness of the feedback presentation.

We will try to help you prepare by providing some general guidelines for giving feedback, discussing how to set treatment goals, and dealing with some of the technical or housekeeping issues included in developing a treatment contact. Our main focus will be the client to whom you offer treatment; however, later in the chapter we will also discuss the feedback process for the client you refuse to treat.

General guidelines for giving feedback

Your feedback to the client lays the foundation for the psychotherapeutic process. You have made a decision that you will offer your client treatment; it is now up to the client to decide whether to accept your assessment of his or her problems and to undertake the course of treatment you have proposed. This must be an informed decision. The client must understand how you perceive the problems, what the goals of treatment will be, what steps may be involved in the treatment process, and the potential risks and gains involved. Without knowledge of all these factors the client cannot make a reasonable decision about progressing with a treatment plan.

Beginners often make the mistake, however, of giving more detail than is necessary or can be usefully assimilated. It is not necessary to relate all your thinking or to try and prove your case. Much of the information that is presented during this interview will subsequently be forgotten or distorted, and there will be other opportunities to review these matters again with your client.

Presenting with authority. The manner in which you provide information to your client is very important. Beginning therapists often have difficulty in presenting material with an air of competence and authority. You may feel unsure of your own judgments and awkward and uncomfortable about presenting your supervisor's ideas. Yet you will need to convince the client that you have a reasonable grasp of the information you are presenting as well as the competence that will allow you to be of assistance.

Your effectiveness will be increased by eliminating the many vague and subjective words or statements that often find their way into the vocabulary of beginners. Such terms as *I think, maybe,* and *sort of* convey uncertainty. There is a considerable difference in impact between saying, "I think this might possibly help you," and saying, "I believe this will be helpful."

In a similar way, beginners detract from their authority and credibility by making discrediting remarks about themselves or their experience, competence, or judgment. The problem is reflected in this therapist's response to a client's question about the success of the proposed treatment: "I am not really sure; I don't have much experience with this, but it may possibly be of help." This statement burdens the client with the therapist's own insecurity and uncertainty. The therapist could be more effective by saying, "Experience shows that this type of approach can be of help and will likely be of assistance to you."

Akin to eliminating vague and discrediting comments is reducing the amount of jargon and technical information you present to your client. Doing this will contribute to a greater sense of shared understanding and greater confidence on the part of the client. Such terms as *agitated depression, obsessiveness,* and *sexual dysfunction* can be confusing and anxiety-producing unless an attempt is carefully made to clarify what these terms mean. Other words, such as *reinforcement, transference,* or *support,* often convey only vague meanings to clients and in fact are not always clearly understood by the beginning therapist. It is very important to use words that are descriptive and meaningful to the client and to be sure that you carefully explain the meaning of any technical language you use.

Strategy. Spending time with your supervisor and reviewing your own material in preparation will both help you gain confidence in what you have to say and give you an opportunity to develop a strategy. Although each situation will warrant individual consideration, it is generally helpful to begin with some restatement of your understanding of the reasons the client has sought treatment; for example: "You have basically come seeking assistance because you have been depressed for over a year and your own efforts have not resulted in much change in your mood." By doing this you start at a point of agreement. You may then advance to presenting your own general impressions of the client's presenting problems, emotional state, and other issues you perceive as important. For example:

My impression coincides with yours in that you seem to have been quite depressed for some time. As a result you have not really been taking good care of yourself and have drifted into general inactivity. Although you haven't presented it in this light, the depression seems to be related to the feelings you have about your marriage and to the sense of not accomplishing some of your major goals.

Broad statements such as these can be given greater clarity and understanding by providing specifics. The seriousness of the depression in the previous example can be underscored by pointing out what the client reported about fatigue, disinterest in eating, and suicidal thinking. The problem suggested about the marriage can be elaborated in terms of the arguments and sexual difficulties described.

In presenting such an overview the beginning therapist often has to discuss problem areas that may not have been identified by the client. For example:

A client came in seeking help with finding an appropriate vocational pursuit. When asked about her marriage during the interview, she suddenly broke into tears. Despite her assertions that she primarily wanted help with her career, she reported a marital crisis that was extremely disturbing to her.

In this situation a beginning therapist may well ask, "Should I present my impression that the marital problem is important and requires attention?" Is it appropriate or even ethical to bring to the client's attention a problem other than that for which he or she has sought help? The difficulty for the therapist is compounded when clients clearly state during the assessment interviews that they do not want to deal with a particular aspect of their life that the therapist comes to see as critical to treatment. For example: A couple sought help for their child because of a learning disability. Almost immediately they asserted that they wanted to help their child but absolutely refused to have anyone meddling in other family problems. Does the therapist who believes that the child cannot be helped without dealing with other family problems state this in the feedback?

We believe it is not only appropriate but necessary that you present your view of the major relevant problems in need of therapeutic intervention, whether or not the client has presented them. In actuality most clients gain confidence in their therapists by recognizing that they are able to perceive aspects of the situation of which they are not aware. On occasion, however, a client may be extremely distressed by having unexpected feedback.

We are not suggesting that every problem that is detected should be part of the feedback. Rather, you should restrict your comments to those issues that are relevant to treatment of the presenting problems, or to those that, although not related, are so critical or compelling that they must be addressed. For example:

> A woman came in for therapy complaining of anxiety symptoms. She reported during the intake inquiry that her four-year-old daughter had not developed speech, but felt that this would come in due course. It seemed to the interviewer that the child's speech problem was not directly related to this woman's focused anxiety symptoms.

In such a case, despite the apparent lack of relevance to the presenting concern, one must bring to the attention of the client the possible seriousness of her daughter's lack of speech.

Providing reassurance. Few clients seek psychotherapeutic assistance without considerable ambivalence about that decision. They may believe that they are not entitled to draw on the help of another person, either because they are not worthy of it or because their problems are not serious enough. Consequently, it is very important to convey to clients for whom you think treatment is appropriate that you view their request as legitimate and reasonable and that you can be, and want to be, of help. It is often useful to say directly, "You have made a good decision to seek help at this time."

The psychotherapist tries to create some feeling of hope. Although you are attempting to set a tone of objectivity with your client, you are also trying to establish a set of some optimism and hope for change. Why should one embark on the often difficult and sometimes painful course of psychotherapy without the expectation that one's life will be bettered in the process? New therapists err on both ends of the continuum of creating a hopeful climate. On one hand, they can neglect to provide the client with clear-cut statements that communicate that some beneficial outcome is likely. It is important to state directly your belief that therapy can be helpful and that the client can derive some important benefits. The therapist can also err, however, by giving the client unrealistic reassurance that things will turn out well. When there is a legitimate source of uncertainty about the outcome, you have the obligation to present it fairly to the client. For example:

> A client with a multiplicity of fears came seeking alleviation of his problems. He made repeated requests for assurance that he could be helped. The therapist told him that systematic desensitization would very likely eliminate his fears.

This example typifies the frequent desire of the beginning therapist to give the client assurance that he will improve and that the treatment being provided will be successful. However, in this case the reassurance was at some cost to objectivity and set the stage for later disappointment and disillusionment with therapy. In addition, such statements detract from the therapist's credibility. The client seeking reassurance often knows how complex and difficult his or her problems are. You should present the potential for gain and also acknowledge the complexity and seriousness of the problems. The therapist in the previous example could have said more effectively:

> You have many serious fears, and some of these may be difficult to alleviate. However, we will be using a treat-

80

ment technique that has often been successful with these types of fears, and I expect you will get some significant relief. We will better know how long treatment might take as we see how therapy progresses.

Giving feedback about testing and consultations

Psychological testing. It can be useful to provide your client with information obtained from psychological testing. Many clients will express an interest in what the tests have shown about them. However, this does not mean the client is requesting or would profit from an in-depth review of the findings as you might explain them to another professional. There is value in making some broad general comments that complement your clinical assessment and add to the client's understanding. Using such information can be particularly helpful in underscoring points of emphasis that support your treatment recommendations. For example:

> The client's psychological evaluation suggested he was a person who had difficulty handling stressful and complex situations. His main coping style was one of avoidance and escape. In giving feedback to the client the therapist used the testing results to point out that the client might well deal with the stresses of therapy by terminating suddenly and prematurely. It was hoped that keeping this concern visible might be a way to prevent such a termination.

Frequently a client who is defensive can better accept information about himself when it is buttressed with testing data that he might see as more factual than interview impressions. For example:

> A client sought help because of his fear that he might kill someone. He was resistant to the idea that his fears might be an overreaction. The psychological testing substantiated the overall clinical impression of an obsessive type of disorder. Information from the evaluation was used to point out that people with this type of testing pat-

81

tern often suffer from fears that they are unlikely to act on. A careful discussion of the test findings helped the man understand and accept that his problem was in his recurrent fears rather than in the risk of his harming someone.

Psychological testing can also provide information about the client's diagnosis. Beginners often wonder if the diagnosis should be reported to the client; this dilemma is heightened when a client directly asks. In general, it is better not to present the client with a formal diagnosis unless there is a compelling reason to do so. It provides little useful information for the client and often conveys meanings that cannot be anticipated and that could be detrimental. In addition, a diagnosis derived solely from psychological testing is open to the inexactness of any isolated score or test. We find it more useful to present the client with some understanding of the diagnostic impression, that is, descriptive information about the type of problem, its severity, and prognosis. For example:

> A man who had recently been hospitalized for an acute but transient psychotic episode asked his therapist what his diagnosis was. The therapist told the client he was diagnosed as schizophrenic, to which the client gave a minimum reply. The therapist did not pursue the matter any further. Following the session the client became increasingly agitated and depressed since he felt that the diagnosis meant he was permanently disabled. Prior to the next therapy session his concerns precipitated a suicide attempt.

In this example the therapist presented a diagnosis that had some meaning to him but conveyed meaning to the client that he did not intend. A formal diagnosis does not appear to have been necessary, but if it was, the therapist should have carefully explained it and explored its impact on the client. He probably would have done better to present a more descriptive diagnostic impression. For example:

You have suffered a brief but very severe emotional reaction during which you were very confused and lost contact with reality. However, you quickly began to improve, and I feel you are now functioning much more effectively. There is every reason to think that your functioning will return to its previous level.

Other consultations. Providing your client with consultative information from other professionals with whom they have had contact is discussed thoroughly in Chapter 5. Although you may find it useful to provide information provided by past therapists, primary care health practitioners, or social service agencies, the implications of sharing this type of information are complex. You should try to limit the information you provide to only that which you believe to be necessary for the client to gain a basic understanding of the situation or that which is necessary for treatment planning.

Setting treatment goals

Developing a set of therapeutic goals is a major step in establishing an alliance between you and your client. Clearly defined goals will provide the client with direction and some means of measuring progress as therapy continues. Your own assessment of appropriate and attainable goals will often mesh with the client's, although they are not likely to be identical or to carry the same priorities. The more your goals differ from the client's, the more discussion and negotiation will be necessary to arrive at a mutually acceptable agreement.

Both your goals and your client's goals will shift and change over the course of therapy. In fact, it is common that after the first six to eight sessions the goals must be reassessed and perhaps new ones established. At this point the client often has received sufficient assistance to reduce the subjective discomfort level of the immediate crisis and must decide whether he or she has further needs for treatment.

During the feedback session you will be presenting the goals you believe should be pursued, the relative priority of each, and the order in which they should be approached. Clients often state their goals in broad, vague ways. The lack of clarity and specificity may be part of the problem the client has in coping with problems. You may make a significant therapeutic contribution by simply stating goals in a concrete, specific manner. For example:

> A client seeking help summed up her complaints by saying, "I want to feel better. I don't want to feel depressed." During the feedback interview the interviewer stated, "An important goal is that you become less depressed. You want to feel happy more of the time, have more energy, see people more frequently, and feel a greater confidence that you can cope with the everyday matters that come your way."

For many people the concept of goals implies long-term, far-reaching matters. Yet your client may be be feeling overwhelmed by the situation and feeling a need for immediate relief. For goals to seem manageable, as well as to provide a sense of accomplishment and movement, they should be relatively short term. Goals can be most meaningful when they have a circumscribed focus and are prescribed in a stepwise fashion, allowing the client to move to new goals as earlier ones are accomplished. For example:

> A client presented his situation as one of nearly complete panic. His wife of twenty years had suddenly left him for another man. He was distraught and repeatedly stated that he did not know what to do. The therapist presented the goals as he saw them, essentially preparing the agenda for therapy. "It is most important that you overcome the panic and depression you are experiencing. You will also have to put your current life in motion again by taking care of your children, maintaining your work, and sustaining your house. Once you have put these things back on some even keel we will take stock of your marital situation and decide what to do with it."

Your ordering of priorities in a useful stepwise approach is the first step in helping the client cope with his or her situation. Knowing what the first step is and not feeling that all goals must be immediately dealt with often will diminish much of the interfering anxiety the client experiences.

Obtaining agreement between you and your client on the goals of therapy is one of the crucial steps in treatment contracting. After presenting the goals it is critical that you actively seek your client's reaction to them and to the proposed order of priority. Although your client may not feel comfortable with what you have suggested, he or she might not say so without some urging from you. In fact, a client may not indicate disagreement until after therapy has proceeded for some time.

Presenting treatment recommendations

Most clients seek therapeutic assistance with very little understanding of what will be involved and have few ideas about what may be asked of them. Their notions about therapy are often laced with misconceptions. Moreover, you may not have a very firm grasp of how therapy will unfold for your client and may find it easy to back away from discussing it in any detail. Yet it is necessary, both from a therapeutic and ethical standpoint, that your clients at least have a skeletal understanding of the treatment approach you plan to offer, the treatment alternatives that exist, what will be expected of them, and what the potential gains and risks might be.

Client expectations. Client's expectations about therapy vary from person to person. Some of these preconceptions may well facilitate your treatment efforts. For example, the client may expect that therapy will be helpful, that responsibilities must be shared, and that solutions are complex and take time. On the other hand, some of the expectations a person brings may interfere with the therapy process – for example, believing that therapy will consist of getting answers to questions, that there will be a mystical transformation imposed by the therapist, or that the act of coming to the therapist's office will result in feeling better. It is useful to be alert to your client's expectations and discuss those that may be counterproductive or unrealistic.

Treatment technique. Describing the treatment in great detail often serves no purpose and can be extremely difficult. However, it is important that the client have some basic idea of what will be happening in the therapy process, what the focus of work will be, and what the shared responsibilities of the client and therapist are. The following are two samples of therapists' descriptions:

> During therapy we will be discussing your concerns about your day-to-day living that you bring to our meetings. That will enable us to focus on those concerns that are most important to you. In the process we will examine how you approach problems, the attitudes you hold, and the feelings you experience. I hope that I will be able to help you examine this material, gain new perspectives on it, and assist you in finding new ways of coping with those areas of your life with which you have difficulty.

> Our major emphasis will be the uncomfortable levels of anxiety that you experience. We will be examining those situations in which you become unduly anxious and the circumstances that trigger it. During our meetings we will basically be working on two major areas. We will be examining the anxiety-producing situations and how you respond, and we will be working with some specific techniques that can help you control anxiety. In addition to coming to the meetings, I will expect you to keep logs on an ongoing basis and to practice some of what you learn here in your daily life.

These examples demonstrate two different approaches to therapy. Your theoretical orientation will always dictate your description of the treatment process. You will note that in both examples the therapist briefly touches on the focus of therapy, the manner in which it will proceed, some expectations for the client, and perhaps to a lesser degree the role of the therapist. Some or all of these points may be expanded.

Treatment alternatives. Sometimes you will select an approach where some clear-cut alternative treatments exist. It is your job to make the decision and choose the approach that you feel will best help your client and fit your skills. However, when there are such clear alternatives, clients should be made aware that there are alternatives, how they would differ from what you propose, and why you have made your particular choice. Again, we are talking basically about presenting the client with a brief synopsis of this issue, not a length discussion. For example:

> A woman sought treatment for her fear of enclosed places. In discussing the proposed treatment the therapist stated, "Basically there are two ways one can treat this type of problem. One method is to try to understand better the reasons you have such fears and attempt to resolve the conflicts that may have caused them. The other, which I am proposing, attempts to help you by lowering the amount of anxiety you feel when you are in such places. The emphasis of our treatment will be the specific problem and symptoms you are experiencing now. We will pay a minimum of attention to the conflicts that may have caused these fears. . . . I am proposing this alternative because it has shown itself to be most effective with cases such as yours and will likely be helpful more rapidly than any other approach."

Gains and risks. In presenting the treatment plan the therapist should also present the gains the client may reasonably expect, as well as the limits of such gains. The latter are less often discussed during treatment contracting, but are equally important. For example, you may expect a client to experience some alleviation of depression

as a result of treatment, but you may also clearly anticipate that there will be times when he or she will again be
depressed. If clients do not understand the limits of treatment, they will not know how to make a realistic assessment of their progress.

A client must also understand any significant risks inherent in the therapeutic venture. Having such an understanding is of importance from a legal as well as an ethical standpoint. If a client of yours suffers some harm
from a risk of which he or she was not informed, you may
be liable for professional malpractice. For example:

> A couple came to a practitioner for marital counseling
> with the hopes that their failing marriage could be saved.
> The wife was at the time involved in an extramarital sex-
> ual relationship. Through the counseling process the wife
> came to believe that she did not want to continue with the
> marriage. A divorce ultimately resulted. At a later time
> the therapist was surprised to find that he was the object
> of a suit. Essentially, the ex-husband was claiming that
> the therapist (and the counseling) was responsible for the
> loss of his wife to another man.

As bizarre as this charge may seem, the failure to have
apprised both members of the obvious risk in counseling
and the limits of assistance placed this professional in a
very difficult position.

It would be foolish to suggest that a client must be apprised of every risk. As in surgery, if a client were to know
every possible low-probability risk, it would be the rare individual who would proceed. We are saying that the client
is entitled to know the *major* risks, which have some significant probability of occurring. One such risk is a probable
negative outcome to therapy. At times you may choose to
offer treatment to a client when in your estimation the
prognosis is poor. However, in such a case you should
clearly state the potential for treatment failure and the
problem that will likely cause the failure. For example:

> A couple requested assistance for sexual problems. It
> was determined by the interviewer that their stormy, cha-

otic relationship would make successful sex treatment un-likely. The couple was told that their propensity to get into frequent destructive fights could well impair their ability to resolve the sexual problem.

Clients whose likelihood of success is poor may be offered treatment when the ongoing risk in the current situation is high and you decide that short-term treatment would probably not have adverse effects. In a sense, one would be saying to the client that, although the prognosis is poor, there is little to lose and something to gain.

Another type of risk is fairly common. In the pursuit of greater well-being, the client may experience uncomfort-able feelings, an exaggeration of symptoms, or new symp-toms. For example:

A man had initiated therapy because of his feelings of dissatisfaction with the way he was running his life. He began to complain in the early sessions that instead of feeling better he was feeling worse. After each meeting he would experience headaches, and prior to sessions would experience high levels of anxiety.

The client, who had been used to avoiding thoughts about his problems, was experiencing the discomfort that comes with focusing on uncomfortable issues. It is not infrequent that a client will terminate early in such a situation because of feeling that therapy is making him or her worse, not better. When you anticipate this reac-tion, it is important to prepare the client for it. The dis-comfort may then be viewed as evidence of progress rather than of failure.

Handling differences of opinion

Most clients, particularly if their subjective discomfort is high, are essentially ready to accept your conceptualiza-tion of their problems and your proposal for treatment. Although it happens only infrequently, beginners often fear that the client will not agree with their impressions and will reject the treatment plan.

If a client seriously questions the treatment proposal, it is essential that you carefully explore his or her reasons before making any decisions about what the next step should be. You must try to understand the client's feelings, motives, and thinking to assess the meaning of the objection. It is often too easy for beginners to question their own judgment and make concessions before the issues are fully explored and understood.

You may well have missed the mark, and careful attention to the client's explanation of his or her complaint may elucidate this for you. However, it is also possible that rejection of your feedback represents some form of resistance or unreasonableness on the part of the client, such as strong needs to control treatment or ambivalence about being in therapy at all. Your judgment concerning the client's complaint will dictate the course of action you take. In some cases you may judge that the differences of opinion result from the failure of the client to understand your recommendations fully. In this instance you would want to reexplain your feedback so that the client clearly understands. This process may take considerable time, but proceeding before you have an agreement is to court premature termination or later problems in therapy.

Other times when your recommendations are challenged you may judge that the client's concern is reasonable and that the matter warrants reconsideration. However, differences will not always be easily negotiable, either because the client's concerns are unreasonable or because there are no other appropriate treatment options. If reexplanation and/or renegotiation are not successful, you may either suggest that the client obtain an independent evaluation of his or her needs or go to another therapist for assistance. In some instances you may make no further recommendation or referral, particularly when you wish to take an extremely strong stand against the specific treatment insisted on by the client. For example:

A man sought treatment for chronic anxiety and his continual preoccupation with feelings of failure. During the initial intake evaluation he mentioned that he hoped he could receive shock treatment so that he would never have to feel bad again. During the feedback the therapist pointed out that such a desire was understandable but unrealistic, and that such treatment would be inappropriate and probably inaccessible to him. An alternative treatment program was recommended. The client refused this, insisting that he wanted shock treatment.

In this case suggesting another helping source was viewed as counterproductive, because the therapist had no reason to believe that any responsible professional would provide this man with shock treatment. The therapist did not wish to lend any credence to his belief that it was obtainable. Instead he continued to emphasize the inappropriateness of the client's desire for this procedure and his unwillingness to provide it. Interestingly enough, in this case the client finally agreed to continue with the treatment recommended.

Handling rejection by the client

Another fear that haunts the student is that the client will decline treatment because of dislike or mistrust of the therapist. Again, this is rare, but when it happens it can be devastating. Beginners tend to react defensively either by arguing or by being overly eager to substitute a new therapist. It is important to remember that this dislike or mistrust on the part of the client does not necessarily reflect on you personally, or on your competence. At this point the client hardly knows you well enough to assess you in either way.

It is more likely that clients will give you critical feedback than refuse to see you altogether. They may express discomfort about you personally, express dissatisfaction with your responses during the session, or possibly raise questions about your competence. The latter issue can be particularly threatening to a student when it focuses on your age, race, sex, student status, or lack of experience — all of which are very sensitive topics. It is important to recognize that, although these concerns may be somewhat reasonable, it is most likely that they are not totally based on objective considerations. For example, if the client questions your credibility, he or she may then be able to discount the importance of threatening comments you make. It may also give the client a feeling of having an edge over you.

When faced with comments of this kind it is a mistake to give immediately and defensively a recitation of your status, experience, qualifications, and the qualifications of your supervisors. Clients who go to a training clinic should know ahead of time that they will be seeing students. If they use that fact to diminish the quality of help they are to receive, they are misusing the situation. When this happens it is most effective to deal with the contradictory aspects of this behavior and the impact their attitudes or concerns may have on therapy itself. It is only after these issues are aired that restating your qualifications becomes useful.

The specter of receiving negative personal feedback from a client can lead a student therapist to avoid discussing the client–therapist relationship. Although you may avoid it initially, strong feelings will ultimately show themselves, and it is better if they are dealt with early in the therapeutic process. You may want to take the opportunity in the feedback process to explore the client's initial feelings toward you as a therapist. In fact, by doing this you indicate to the client that his or her feelings about you and the therapeutic relationship are matters to be openly discussed. It is a good idea to ask the client toward the end of the interview "How did you feel talking to me today?" or, "What were your reactions to today's meeting?"

There will be times when the client's rejection of the therapist will require a change in therapist. As we have pointed out, the client does have the right ultimately to choose whom he will see, although the facility has the right to decide whether it will provide service to that person on that basis. It is hard to set up guidelines for such decisions. Changing therapists makes the most sense when the client obviously needs assistance, when he or she is adamantly opposed to the therapist, and when the complaint is tied to a specific quality that is unlikely to reoccur with another therapist.

However, such a decision has important therapeutic implications that warrant further investigation and clarification. Any change of therapist at this point should be viewed as a serious change in therapeutic plans and should be carefully reviewed by you and your supervisor.

Agreeing to a treatment contract

After you have presented your impressions, it is now up to the client to decide whether to accept what you have said and agree to proceed with treatment. Prior to raising that question directly, you should leave some time to obtain any reactions or concerns the client may have had about the material you have presented. This is one of many points where you must carefully check with your client to get reactions and to be sure you have been understood.

Most clients at this point are ready to make an affirmative decision about continuing with treatment. However, some may want more time to think about the decision. Given a significant degree of uncertainty or ambivalence, it is generally better to have the client return after having had time to consider it than to press for an immediate decision or to leave the answer to a telephone contact. A face-to-face contact is more likely to lead to an affirmative decision and allows you to deal personally with any fears, concerns, or misconceptions that arise.

Once the client has agreed to continue in treatment,

there still remains an array of important "housekeeping" or technical considerations that you need to cover before proceeding with therapy. Although less substantive, they are of nearly equal importance to the previous topics and issues you have covered with your client. These include the variety of parameters within which therapy will proceed, such as scheduling and length of sessions, duration of therapy, fees, and termination.

Sessions. It is of course important that your client know when and where your sessions will be held, what the frequency of meetings will be, and the length of each meeting. New therapists are often lackadaisical about the length of treatment interviews. We believe it is important generally to hold to the allocated time, unless the particular type of therapy being used demands flexibility. Having a consistent amount of time provides a useful structure for both you and your client and permits each person to pace himself accordingly.

The setting of appointment times is often viewed as perfunctory. However, the sheer amount of material that the client has had to assimilate and his or her level of anxiety often result in errors in recall about appointments. Once a mutually agreeable time is set it can be extremely helpful to write it down and hand it to the client rather than to rely on a verbal understanding.

Missed appointments. Some clients will view the appointments in a casual way, whereas others will see them as inviolate. Given this array of attitudes about time commitments and toward therapy in general, it is useful to convey that the time established is being set aside for the client, and it is expected that he or she will make the arrangements necessary to keep the appointment. Clients should understand that if they cannot keep the appointment, it is their responsibility to notify the therapist and set up another time. Often this approach appears rather inflexible and perhaps trivial to the new therapist until he or she has a client who fails to keep several appointments. Such occurrences can be extremely frustrating and angering. Similarly you will want your client to be on time. Again, some people are consistently responsible and others chronically late. Although students often prefer a more informal contract, it is useful to end the meeting at the regular time, regardless of the client's time of arrival. This essentially conveys that they have a particular meeting time for which they are held responsible. There are, of course, always exceptions to such rules, as in the case of an infrequent inadvertent lateness or emergencies.

Fees. Although not all training clinics charge fees, there may well be a fee involved for treatment, often one based on ability to pay. It is necessary that the client know his or her financial obligations at this initial contracting meeting (i.e., how much treatment will cost and how payment is expected). In many ways this is the most difficult of the housekeeping issues for students. First, money is one of the most difficult topics to discuss in our culture. Second, the payment of a fee implies that the client will be getting something of worth in return, and beginning therapists often question whether their service is worth the fee charged. Lastly, there seems to be an attitude among those pursuing the mental health professions that makes it difficult to charge for assistance.

As a result of these varied issues, the student often tries to deal with the topic of fees in a perfunctory manner. He or she may treat it as an annoyance imposed by the institution, and form an alliance with the client by establishing an unrealistically low fee. Because the matter of charging fees is such a sensitive one, it is important that the student therapist grapple with his or her own feelings and biases and deal with the client in a sensitive, thoughtful, and fair manner. Setting fees provides an opportunity to learn more about your client – his or her financial situation, attitudes about money, and ways of managing resources. You will also gain information about how your client sets priorities and organizes his or her life.

In establishing the fee it is important to find out what this expenditure of money will mean to the client and what problems it will create. It is equally important to ascertain how the client feels about paying the fee. Some people who can afford a fee may resent it, despite its size. There is a tendency for students to "oil the squeaky wheel" and establish the lowest fees for the clients who complain the most. The result is often inequitable for those who accept the fee although they may be no more able to pay it than those who complain. In general, the most equitable fee structure is one that is fairly applied to all.

Refusing to treat the client

Thus far the focus of this chapter has been the client to whom you offer therapy. Now we turn to the client to whom you refuse treatment. In this situation the feedback session takes on even greater importance, because it may be the last time you meet with the client. It is critically important to clarify the issues or misunderstandings, particularly because the circumstances that result in your declining to offer treatment often include a great likelihood of misunderstanding and distortion. For these reasons precise communication is exceedingly important.

There could be any number of reasons for refusing treatment: The service necessary may not be available at your facility, the person may require a more experienced therapist, or there may be some contingencies such as hospitalization or medication, that might make it advisable to handle the case elsewhere. Although such situations may seem fairly straightforward on the surface, the denying of treatment or referral for any reason can be very troublesome. Seeking treatment is generally a major step; now the client must again initiate this process and again try to explain his or her problems and concerns to another therapist.

Although you may perceive the referral as acting in the client's best interests, the client may well perceive the denial of immediate treatment as a personal rejection or an indication that you do not see him or her as worthy or capable of being helped. The problematic nature of this situation is reflected in the relatively low number of referred patients who follow through and successfully obtain therapy elsewhere.

You cannot completely avoid these problems, but you can minimize them by carefully communicating the reasons that treatment is not being offered, acknowledging the fears and concerns the client may have, checking for distortion and clarifying any misconceptions, and facilitating the referral in an active way.

The referral process itself is crucial. Too frequently once the referral is made the burden of responsibility is left to the client. If the therapist takes an active, facilitating role, the likelihood of a success is much greater. This can be accomplished by giving the client some specific places to go to get appropriate treatment. You will need to know ahead of time those persons or institutions that are willing and able to offer the service needed. Otherwise the client may well be turned away again. In addition, the client must know how to contact the new facility and where it is located. Many clients are overwhelmed by the ambiguity of an unknown place. The likelihood of a successful referral is greatly increased when the party to whom the client is referred knows something about the referral and expects a contact from your client. This decreases the possibility of confusion when the client makes the contact. Finally, the referral route can be long and arduous; the client may have to wait to be seen. You can best serve your client by maintaining contact until he or she is seen by the new therapist. This may only be by telephone, but it limits the likelihood of the client despairing and giving up.

Ending the feedback session

Considering the many topics you will need to cover in the feedback and contracting session, you may well find yourself running short of time. It is important, however, to leave some time at the end of the session, even if that requires leaving some housekeeping issues for the next session. This time allows you to solicit once again any reactions to the session or questions that still remain unanswered. These need not necessarily be dealt with in this session, but can become part of the agenda for the next meeting.

Lastly, it will be helpful to summarize briefly and establish a focus for the next meeting. Therapists tend to forget that the client needs to feel he has received something of value from this series of evaluations and feedback meetings, whether this be new understanding of himself, some new directions, or hope for the future.

8

Conducting the session

The shift from a relatively structured information-gathering situation to the less predictable and more complex therapy interaction often causes the student therapist considerable anxiety. Lacking immediate and limited goals that were present for the initial interviews, you may find yourself at a loss as to what to do. It is difficult to make the transition from interviewer to therapist. The roles may demand very different and often contradictory behavior from you.

In an effort to cope with this bewildering situation, many beginning therapists will cling to a "do-something" orientation: asking a question, giving advice, offering the client alternatives, changing the subject – anything that will get things moving.

The process of therapy is not an experience in which one person does something *to* another. It is a complex interaction between two or more people with the ultimate goal of facilitating some beneficial and, it is hoped, long-term changes in the client. The effects of treatment are seldom seen immediately, and, as a result, students commonly feel frustrated and discouraged. The situation will become less stressful for you if you can abandon the "cure" and "do-something" orientation and avoid focusing on your need to accomplish some measurable change within each hour.

Another source of anxiety for students at this point is the fear of missing something or of not responding appropriately to some issue your client brings up. It is unlikely that any beginning therapist will be capable of dealing with all material equally effectively. To do so requires a variety of skills that can be mastered only after a great deal of experience. Remember that most truly important issues in therapy will be brought up repeatedly. As you learn more about your client you will become increasingly able to recognize relevant issues and to respond therapeutically.

The varied and subtle nature of the therapy interaction makes it difficult to prescribe specific rules for conducting a therapy session. We cannot specify how to conduct your sessions in the same manner that we described how to conduct an intake interview. What you ultimately decide to do within the hour is affected by a variety of interacting factors. Each therapist will follow some relatively unique pattern, which is dictated by (1) his or her therapeutic orientation, available skills, and personality; (2) the specific treatment goals; and (3) the characteristics of the individual client. Although one's therapeutic orientation will provide some guidance, each therapist will vary the strategy to suit his or her personal style and the response of the particular client. To be effective you must be flexible and responsive to how the client reacts to your approach and the techniques you are using.

There are some fundamental tools that are widely applicable across theoretical frameworks and that will be useful in conducting your therapy sessions. However, the general guidelines that follow will have to be supplemented by direct supervision and more detailed reading about specific treatment approaches.

How to begin a session

You may choose from three general approaches when beginning a therapy session. One option is simply to say nothing, although this alternative is often forgotten when a student therapist is feeling anxious in the first minutes of a session. It gives the client the opportunity to let you know immediately what may be on his or her mind.

There are times when silence is the best approach. This is particularly true when you have been seeing a client for some time and are fairly comfortable with one another. In such situations your silence can help to draw out new and productive material without your being a guiding influence. Alternatively, you may choose to remain silent to force a client who tends to be overly dependent on you to initiate discussion.

There are some potential hazards in using this approach, however. If you are not skilled at asserting yourself, it is quite possible that a talkative, forceful client will take your silence as a cue to dominate the session. On the other hand, if your client is apprehensive and unsure about what is going to happen, your silence may increase his or her anxiety.

A second alternative is for the therapist to pose an open-ended, nondirective question, such as, "How have things been going for you this week?" or, "How have you been feeling since we last met?" or, "What would you like to work on today?" We think that this alternative is the appropriate choice for most clients. It has the value of giving the client permission to bring up pressing concerns that may need attention while at the same time providing some guidance to help him or her focus on what is important.

The third option for beginning a session is to ask a more specific question referring to some issue brought up in the previous session or to a between-session homework assignment. Such questions as, "Last week we were talking about. . . . Have you given that any more thought?" or, "What was your experience like when you tried . . . ?" fit into this category. This approach immediately places responsibility for directing the session clearly in your hands. It has drawbacks, however, because you may miss the opportunity to pick up on pressing issues that may be unrelated to your question.

101

Although there may be certain issues you wish to discuss during a session, much can be gained by checking with the client before getting to specifics. For example: "I'd really like to talk to you about the issue we were dealing with last week, but first I'd like to find out how things have been going for you. Is there anything pressing you'd like to discuss first?" In practice you may well find that what works best for you will be a combination of the approaches discussed. You may begin by sitting down with the client, pausing, and allowing him or her to bring up spontaneously anything that may be pressing. If nothing emerges, you can then pose some sort of open-ended question and eventually become more specific if desired.

Whatever approach you select, it is always important to assess the affect and mood of your client for indications on how to proceed. Does the client have a smile on his or her face and seem excited about beginning therapy? Is he or she anxious, looking around the room, avoiding your gaze, or fidgeting in the chair? Are there any physical signs of change in the individual's manner of dressing, general grooming, or manner of walking? All this information gives you a basis for making judgments on how to adjust your style and in what direction to proceed.

There may be times when a client begins the hour with a statement like, "I don't have much to say today," or, "You talk today, I don't know what to talk about." This is another dilemma for the beginner. You must learn how to interpret the meaning of such a remark in order to know how to respond. Is the client really blocking and unable to think of anything to say? Is he or she trying to avoid some topic or area of difficulty? Is he or she angry with you? These may all be possibilities. Your knowledge of your client as well as the emotion evident in the interaction will help you decide this question. For example, if you think the client is likely to be avoiding an anxiety-provoking topic that was discussed last session, you might ask, "How did you respond to last week's session?"

If you lack an immediate hypothesis, you may simply decide to respond directly to the face value of the client's statement and make a general opening remark, such as, "Tell me what has been happening this past week." This latter option could help a genuinely blocking client to produce some material for discussion.

Facilitating and focusing discussion

One of your major tasks as a therapist will be to encourage focused discussion of issues that bear on the therapy goals. Some clients can be depended on spontaneously to open discussion on areas important to treatment, which will make your job far easier. Others, however, pose problems by either talking too much or too little.

The client who sits silently and responds to your questions with monosyllabic answers seems to the most troublesome of the two extremes for beginners. Students tend to feel quite uncomfortable about sitting in silence and often take the responsibility for a topic to discuss. This tactic is rarely successful, because the more you talk, the more silent the client is likely to become.

Many of the suggestions we made in reference to handling the anxieties of the initial interview are helpful when you are trying to elicit relevant therapeutic material from a client. An individual who has sought the help of a therapist usually feels considerable apprehension about actually delving into the most pertinent issues. In order for your client to become more comfortable with the process of therapy, you must be patient, supportive, and empathetic. You will probably also have to learn to tolerate some silences. Yet you must also be firm and clear in communicating the expectation that the client shares the responsibility for generating relevant discussion, however difficult that may be. Patience and persistence are the key qualities for the therapist in these situations. It is also helpful to remember to initiate questioning in a broad, open-ended fashion, because you are likely to get brief, unproductive answers in response to specific questions.

There may be times when patience, support, and open-ended probing have little effect on the client's reticence to discuss his or her problems. In these instances it may be necessary for you to confront the client directly with his or her lack of participation and its negative consequences before any of the work of therapy can actually begin.

Other clients, however, will deluge you with a range of matters, some or most of which may be inconsequential to therapy. Your problem will then be one of controlling the discussion and directing it into clinically relevant areas. Beginners commonly respond to their fear of missing something important by attempting to pursue every idea the client mentions. This tactic is generally unproductive, because it does not allow time to follow up any one area in sufficient depth.

However, students have difficulty sifting through and deciding what is fruitful to develop and what to allow to pass without further discussion. These decisions about the clinical importance of topics are dictated in large part by the goals of therapy and by your choice of treatment approach. However, we can offer some general guidelines that apply to most situations.

A topic must be dealt with in some way if a client repeatedly brings it up as a matter of concern, even if you do not judge it particularly relevant to the treatment. You must be responsive to the client's needs to talk about certain issues, yet you must also try to educate him or her about the most profitable way to approach discussion of the problem. For example:

> A young woman client entered therapy with the presenting problems of anxiety and depression about her job. After gathering information about the client and her problem situation, the therapist and client agreed that her current problems related to long-standing interpersonal difficulties with authority figures in her life.

104

During the first therapy session the client complained extensively about the working conditions of her job. The therapist was supportive and allowed her to discuss her work environment rather than her relationships. The second interview began in the same vein; however, this time the therapist responded differently, saying, "I recognize that there are many things about your job that are unsatisfactory to you. Your relationships at work must contribute in large part to that dissatisfaction. I think it would be most profitable for us to begin to examine those relationships. What do you think about that idea?"

Here the therapist was supportive of the client's wish to discuss matters of concern to her but at the same time directed her attention to a more therapeutically fruitful area. Note that the therapist specifically asked for the client's reaction to the idea instead of abruptly redirecting the conversation.

The level of anxiety or degree of emotion that a client displays when discussing a given topic may also be indicative of its importance as a treatment issue. In general, you may view anxiety or a strong emotional reaction to a subject as evidence that it is troublesome to the client in some way. On the other hand, it is also significant when an individual who is discussing a topic or situation that would normally elicit an emotional reaction shows little or no effect.

Not all clients will give you equally reliable indicators of their level of discomfort. There are individuals whose pattern is to be glib and flatly unemotional about all topics and who show little overt sign of anxiety. With such people it is generally wise to focus on subject matter that is most obviously related to the treatment goals and to follow up persistently on any evidence of inconsistency and discomfort.

There are clients at the opposite extreme, who typically react with overconcern to a wide range of situations and whose overt anxiety offers you little in terms of differentiating significant topics. Such people will perhaps respond to a calm and reassuring therapeutic style accompanied by considerable guidance to help them focus on the more productive issues.

Pursuing relevant topics

Exploring the dimensions of an issue. We have discussed some ways of assessing a topic with regard to its value as a treatment issue. Once you make the initial judgment to pursue an area in therapy you will need to explore it further in order to determine the degree and kind of significance it holds for your client. For example, how far-reaching is the issue? Does it have broad or very specific ramifications? Is it an example of a troublesome pattern or only an isolated incident? What is the degree of feeling or discomfort associated with it? What are its implications or consequences? How does it relate to the problems the client is having in daily life and/or in therapy? We can outline some tools that may be useful in evaluating these dimensions. Once again, however, these should be seen as general suggestions that will be modified according to your theoretical approach.

By questioning and guiding your client you can pursue a feeling, thought, or behavior in sufficient depth that it becomes clear to both of you how it relates to the behavioral pattern you are both working to change. Ideally, your questions should be based on some hypothesis you have about how the issue is related to one or more of the therapeutic concerns that have emerged. Therapeutic questions are not based on curiosity or asked purely out of desire for more information; rather, their intent is to help clarify for both of you the client's experience, thoughts, and feelings.

Assume, for example, that you are treating a man who is depressed. You believe his depression is related to his difficulty in effectively asserting his rights in interpersonal conflict situations. The overall goal with this client, then, is to teach him assertion skills. The client begins a session by telling you that he is getting bored with his job. Keeping your goals in mind, you may use the situation to draw out information about the interpersonal interactions he experiences at work. It may be that recurring incidents of his acting unassertively are contributing to his feeling of boredom. Another tactic that could be used in the same situation is to question the client about the feeling of boredom – what it is like, what other situations seem to elicit it, and when he is more or less bored. Both of these approaches could lead into exploring the client's unassertive behavior.

Another technique that is helpful in gaining a clearer understanding of the dimensions of a specific issue is to rephrase in your own words what you have heard. Such a restatement provides an opportunity for both of you to check out your assumptions and to reach a mutual understanding. For example, a client began the session stating: "Every time I think about my problem I can think of ten different ways to deal with it and I can't decide what to do." The therapist clarified the client's statement by rephrasing it in this way: "You are having trouble thinking and having difficulty making decisions."

If you have some personal reactions or speculations about how the incident connects with broader patterns in your client's life, you may present those to him or her as hypotheses: "It seems to me that this relates to that pattern we have discussed before . . . your tendency to avoid conflict situations and to try to placate your friends. Do you see a connection?" or, "I have a hypothesis about how this relates to another problem we have discussed . . . What do you think?" Statements of this type allow you to present your thoughts and at the same time enlist your client's help in drawing a conclusion.

There are times when such tactics will not be sufficient to help your client to recognize significant patterns that are counterproductive. In order to be effective in these situations you may need to challenge what your client says or believes. To use confrontation well you must be willing to deal with negative reactions from the client. You must also feel fairly confident about your own judgment, which is particularly difficult when your client disagrees with you. This is a situation where students become extremely uncomfortable. Trusting your reaction to something your client says or does takes experience; building that experience requires a willingness to take some calculated risks. We will discuss in more depth in the next chapter how to assess your relationship with a client and how to use confrontation.

Questioning, giving feedback, offering hypotheses, drawing connections, and confronting are all basic tools to help you pursue a topic therapeutically. These techniques will assist you both in exploring the dimensions and relevance of an issue as well as in working with the problem to bring about change. There are a variety of other responses available to you, and again your choices will depend on your treatment strategy and goals. We cannot discuss all the possibilities in depth in this book; however, by mentioning some of them we hope to raise your awareness of the broad range and variety of responses available.

For example, you may choose to offer your client advice, give support, provide information, or teach skills. You may encourage self-expression, new behaviors, different ways of viewing the world, risk taking, and change. You may deliberately withhold your reaction to what the client is saying or doing, or you may respond with praise or criticism. Therapists both help clients to become aware of their feelings and ignore their feelings, depending on the situation and the client.

What is striking in listing some of the possibilities is that the responses you select to help one client will be totally inappropriate to the next. What you do one session may need to be altered the next time you meet. It is critical to be broadly skilled in a variety of techniques so that you will be able to modify your therapeutic style to suit the variety of situations you will encounter in clinical practice.

Choice of strategy. For beginners it is useful to make two very broad distinctions about how to approach therapy with a client. These distinctions do not do justice to the complexity and subtlety of therapeutic strategy, nor do they differentiate the fine points of theoretical methodologies. However, they are helpful to students in terms of giving them ways of conceptualizing *what to do* in a therapy session.

Generally your choice of therapeutic strategy, whatever its theoretical origins, may be viewed in one of two ways: either you will focus on one problem area to the exclusion of other topics of possible concern, or you will broadly scan your discussions with the client to isolate recurring themes or patterns and develop several problem areas simultaneously. For example, therapists treating clients for sexual dysfunction or deviations, specific fears, obesity, or alcoholism will typically inattend to evidence of other problem areas unless they interfere with the progress of therapy. This extremely focused approach would be less appropriate, for instance, with an individual complaining of chronic depression who cannot isolate specific difficulties. For such a person it would be more useful initially to examine a broad spectrum of concerns and gradually to focus on a few recurring themes that might bear on the problems, such as difficulty with assertiveness or an overwhelming sense of responsibility for others. For other clients you may alternate your strategy, moving from the broad-based to the problem-focused, depending on your judgment at the time about what would be most useful.

Evaluating progress. Students often have difficulty in making a judgment about when they are finished working with an issue. You rarely actually finish discussing a topic. Most issues can be explored on many levels and still provide therapeutic material. As the process of therapy proceeds, you will find that subjects discussed several weeks ago come up in a different light and can be pursued again in a different way. It is helpful to recognize that discussion of any given issue is rarely completed but, rather, is interrupted for periods of time only to emerge again as part of a general theme or pattern.

People are capable of absorbing various amounts of input at a given time. You will gradually learn to assess how much each client is able to attend to in one session. By being sensitive to signs of the client's anxiety, anger, or boredom you will learn to judge when your efforts have ceased to be useful. This again is a stylistic difference among people that can only be evaluated on an individual basis. Viewing video tapes or listening to audio tapes of sessions will be invaluable in helping you to pick up such cues.

Shifting the focus of your discussion from one topic to another is an important skill that requires practice. When you feel that a given area has been discussed to the limit of its usefulness, it is helpful to make some closing summary statement to facilitate shifting focus. For example: "Let's see what happens and we'll talk about it again," or, "I don't feel there's much value in pursuing this issue further right now. We'll look at it later." Once the topic is temporarily closed, you are at a choice point, much as you were at the beginning of the hour. You can remain silent and allow your client to bring up another topic, or you can initiate discussion of a specific point you wish to pursue. There is also the option at this time of looking at a different aspect of the same topic you have been discussing. The skills of appropriate timing and graceful bridging from one topic to another are ones that will take a great deal of time to develop.

It is often difficult for students to appreciate that the continual repetition of major points is often necessary. It may seem as though you have said the same thing a dozen times before your client has demonstrated that he or she understands and can use it. This can be frustrating experience, particularly when you view your client's behavior as self-destructive or clearly counterproductive.

It is important to remember that those patterns of behavior for which your clients are seeking help may be long-standing and have become troublesome because clients have been unable to change them on their own. Therefore it is to be expected that an understanding and altering of these patterns will take time.

There will be some clients for whom progress will be rapid and visible. As we have pointed out before, people in acute distress often feel better after one interview and even within a single session may demonstrate a change in outlook. On the other hand, there are people whose ambivalence about change will hamper their progress to such an extent that you may never feel that you are getting closer to your goal. You may be tempted to terminate a client when you feel that you are getting nowhere. However, a judgment such as this should be carefully thought out and thoroughly discussed with your supervisor. This issue is developed more fully in the chapter dealing with termination.

How to end a session

The ending of a session is rarely planned or even given much thought ahead of time. Students often view the conclusion of a session as something that just happens when the hour is up. As with all aspects of conducting a therapy session, a graceful conclusion requires skill.

The manner in which an hour ends can be quite significant in terms of its effect on future sessions. If your client feels abruptly cut off at the end of an hour, you may undermine all your previous efforts to create an accepting and supportive atmosphere. On the other hand, if you allow a client to continue talking well past the end of the hour, he or she may come to believe that the formal structure of therapy can be manipulated at will. At either extreme, a poor ending can be detrimental to the progress of treatment.

Planning ahead in preparing for the end of the session is

very important. Being aware of how much time is left is crucial to prevent having to cut your client off abruptly. A major part of keeping control of a session is being well aware of the time restrictions and not allowing your client to get involved in a highly emotional issue just minutes before the end of a session. There will doubtless be times when you will have to cut a client off, particularly if he or she is very talkative. You should be aware of when and why you are doing this, however, and weigh the potential consequences carefully.

Students are often thrown off guard by clients who discuss relatively inconsequential things for most of the hour and then repeatedly bring up a very important issue at the end, hoping to gain control and hold the therapist's attention for a longer time. With such clients it is particularly important to stay within the time limits and maintain your control. Saying something like, "This is a very important point; let's discuss it at the beginning of our next session," or, "I wish you had brought this up earlier since our time is up now; be sure to mention it next week," will help minimize this sort of problem.

You may want to conclude your session with some sort of summarizing statement or specific instruction for what you want your client to do between sessions. The end of the session also provides you with an opportunity to reiterate a point that you feel is particularly important or to voice some specific reaction to the hour. You may also choose to set the stage for the next session by briefly mentioning some area you will want to cover. If you choose this alternative, or the one of giving a specific "homework" assignment, it is important that you remember to refer to these items in the next session. It can be very distressing for a client to work on an assignment for a week only to find that it is not mentioned in the next session. Such an experience can greatly hamper your credibility and effectiveness.

In summary, when you near the end of a session you should be aware of the time and make an effort to reach some closure before the time is up. Be prepared with a closing phrase, such as, "Our time is up for today," or, "We will need to end now"; then check to be sure that the client is finished and that another appointment is scheduled. Clients may react very differently to your efforts to conclude a session. Again, you will find it necessary to modify your style for each individual while maintaining sufficient control to end within reasonable time limits.

9

Some more sophisticated therapy skills

In previous chapters we have discussed primarily the skills involved in dealing with the content of a therapy session. However, the interaction between therapist and client has a far more complex structure than the surface content of a therapeutic hour might imply. We find it useful in training beginning students to view this complexity in terms of content versus process. By *content* we refer to the overt substance of the topics being discussed. The term *process* refers to the *way* the client presents himself or herself and the problems to you as well as the stages through which therapy progresses.

The process aspects of the therapeutic hour include longitudinal variables, such as the quality and nature of the relationship between client and therapist and the patterns of the client's problem-solving attempts over time. They also involve more immediate factors, such as what the client says versus what is omitted, how it is said, and what is communicated nonverbally. These are the concepts we will introduce in this chapter. We have chosen to talk about them in terms of levels of interaction, with the higher levels being further removed from the surface content of the client's statements and requiring simultaneous consideration of complex aspects of the therapy hour.

Any attempt at a clear distinction between the process and the content of therapy is by nature artificial. Yet we find that viewing these aspects as separate can be helpful in the process of teaching therapy skills. As you read this chapter you will find that certain points will have clear meaning for you, and you will be able to translate them into action in your ongoing therapy contacts. Other points, however, will seem vague, obscure, or not immediately applicable to your level of learning. We're not making an effort here to delineate the details of how one becomes more advanced as a therapist. This goes hand in hand with developing a more specialized theoretical perspective, which we have not addressed here. We can, however, attempt to point out issues that add increased complexity to the therapy experience for you and your client. As your amount of experience as a therapist increases, points mentioned in this chapter that may seem obscure to you now will become increasingly meaningful.

Levels of the psychotherapeutic interaction

First level. The first concerns of a beginning therapist generally center around the content of the material the client brings up in a session. This is the most obvious and "safest" therapeutic material to comment on. Needless to say, this focus is necessary in order to allow the therapist to assess what is happening in the client's life and how the client views his or her problems. We shall consider this focus on content the first level for the purpose of clarifying the different levels of interaction in the therapeutic process.

Focusing on content allows you to gain information efficiently about specific incidents, problems, or reactions your client has experienced. This focus is of limited value, however, when it is the only material being considered by the therapist. If you deal strictly with the content of what your client reports, your understanding of that material is limited to what your client sees as problematic and furthermore to the portion of the problem that he or she can recognize. An example may help to make this point clearer:

A twenty-three-year-old obese man has sought therapy to help him deal with a number of problem areas, which include his obesity and depression. The therapist has seen him for several weeks and offered him a number of behavioral suggestions to help him gain some control over his weight and decrease his depression. This client had attempted to follow each new program but was unable to pursue any one for more than a few days. He began the session by telling the therapist, "I have decided that all my other problems are just a result of my weight, so I'm considering having my jaw wired shut. That will *make* me lose weight. What do you think of that idea?" The student therapist was surprised by this announcement and chose to deal only with the content of his statement. He responded, "That will depend. What do you know about the procedure? What are its advantages and disadvantages in your eyes?"

Consider what the therapist in this example said. You may well feel that in the same situation your response would have been similar. Beginning therapists typically do find it easiest to deal with the content of the client's statement. The anxiety and pressure to come up with a useful response can add to the tendency to stay at the content level. It takes more time, more thought, and a broader base of experience to view a situation from a different perspective. With increased experience you will learn to trust your own reactions to what is going on, in addition to the surface content as your client presents it.

Second level. During the process of therapy the client provides the therapist with direct exposure to his or her problem-solving style. Viewing your client's behavior in therapy as a sample of the person's general behavior outside that context requires a more complex type of analysis. If he had been able to readjust his focus a bit, the therapist in the preceding example might well have seen his client's suggestion as relevant to some broader therapeutic issue. Another therapist might have dealt with this same client by responding to this more complex level of analysis in the following way:

Client: I'm considering having my jaw wired shut. That will *make* me lose weight. What do you think of that idea?

Therapist: Well I don't know. That is reminiscent of a way of dealing with problems that I've seen you use before. You tend to look for a solution that won't require you to change your behavior.

By attending to recurring behavior patterns this therapist has become aware of a stylistic approach to problems that interferes with his client's efforts to change. He used this information as a basis for providing feedback to the client that was relevant to an issue far broader than the immediate situation raised by the client.

As you become more aware of the multiple levels of interaction in the therapeutic exchange, you will also find yourself making increasingly complex judgments about how and when to respond. The issues that should be considered as you make these judgments will become clearer to you as we proceed and as you gain experience.

Third level. As we have mentioned repeatedly, psychotherapy takes place in the context of an interpersonal relationship. You and your client will affect one another as people, and the psychotherapeutic situation can be viewed as an arena for observing how your client relates interpersonally. Granted, the "doctor-patient" characteristics of this relationship make it different in many ways from more typical interactions between people. Nevertheless, you have a very real sample of how your client deals with interpersonal relationships when you analyze the therapy interaction from this perspective.

Does it appear that the client is always making an effort to please you and to gain your approval regardless of the cost to him or her? Does he or she seem to resist efforts on your part to offer support or empathy by discounting your statements with such phrases as "You don't understand"? Does your client debate or argue about every point you discuss in an effort to prove you wrong? There are, of course, a multitude of ways of relating, and the character of any given therapeutic relationship will change over time.

Being aware of how your actions are likely to affect your client gives you a significant advantage in creating an approach that is most likely to produce change in the desired direction. For example, when a client consistently responds to supportive gestures from the therapist by discounting that support and accusing the therapist of not understanding, continued efforts in the same vein would most likely not be profitable.

Using this added dimension to develop a response, another therapist may have dealt with the jaw-wiring proposal in this way:

> Client: What do you think of that idea?
> Therapist: In the past you have asked for my advice and then rejected it, saying that my suggestions didn't work for you. This makes me reluctant to offer my opinion now. It also reminds me of some similar situations you've described with your last boss. Do you see any connection?

There are, of course, many ways in which a therapist can use this level of analysis to facilitate treatment. It is particularly useful for clients whose problems revolve around interpersonal relating. As illustrated in the last example, the therapeutic relationship can be seen as an arena in which you can directly experience and examine the client's troublesome interpersonal style. There is a great advantage to focusing on this level, because you may be able to correct the blind spots in the client's awareness of how he or she affects other people.

This dimension of the therapeutic process is a highly complex one. You may find yourself aware of a pattern in your client's response to your behavior but unable to decide how to deal with it. There is seldom a clear right or wrong approach at this level.

Fourth level. The view of therapy as an interaction between people implies that just as your behavior affects your client, his or her behavior affects you. Acknowledging your personal reactions to a client's behavior and using them to reach the therapy goals adds a fourth component to the complex process of developing a therapeutic response.

Put yourself in the position of a therapist in our example. How do you imagine you might feel? It is entirely possible that you would be frustrated or even angry. You may have put a lot of effort into developing a number of carefully considered programs to help the client. The fact that he has repeatedly failed to hold up his part of the bargain is certainly cause for frustration and disappointment. Now he presents you with an alternative that requires no effort on his part, rejecting your efforts to help him.

A therapist might voice a direct personal reaction to the client in order to help him become more aware of how his behavior affects others. For example:

> You know, I'm feeling awfully frustrated and annoyed right now. As I see it, we agreed that I would help you find ways to change. You've repeatedly rejected my suggestions, and I really don't think you're holding up your part of the bargain.

Assessing your own emotional reaction may be just the starting point for formulating a response. Once you have acknowledged your feelings to yourself, you can use this information to help you analyze what is happening between you and your client. Why is this behavior by your client so frustrating and angering to you? There are a number of issues to consider in answering this question. You need to determine what aspects of your client's behavior you are responding to. You may decide that your reaction has more to do with *you* than with the client. For example, you may be angry with the client for making you feel like a failure. This is a common reaction for beginners when their clients do not make progress as quickly as they'd like. In this case you would probably not base an intervention in therapy on these feelings, but rather add them to your growing knowledge about your own idiosyncratic responses to doing therapy. You must ask yourself whether your reactions or the client's behavior in question are relevant to reaching the goals of therapy. This is really the determining factor for deciding how and when to use your personal feelings.

For example, another therapist might have viewed this same set of events quite differently. Acknowledging that this client's suggestion has made him angry and frustrated, he considers what has led to these feelings. Perhaps he has taken too much responsibility for finding a solution to the problems and has allowed the client to make a minimum investment of effort in the process of change. The therapist considers all this information in formulating a response:

> Client: What do you think of that idea?
> Therapist: Of course, such an operation is an alternative that has always been available to you. If you decide to take that route, that decision will be entirely your own. I will take no part in it. You and I have embarked on this therapy in an effort to help you change some self-destructive behavior patterns, and I have presented several alternative ways for you to begin those changes. You have told me that none of these methods have worked for you. It seems to me that you are refusing to take responsibility for changing yourself.

One note of caution: Using your own emotional reactions to clients as a basis for therapeutic interventions can be an extremely powerful tool. Just as the client introduces his or her own characteristic style and personal problems into the therapeutic relationship, so may the therapist. It is very important that you avoid projecting your own problems onto the client. We recommend using this level of analysis only after careful consideration.

Although a few students make the mistake of too quickly attributing their own idiosyncratic responses to their clients, most students err in the opposite direction. In order to operate at this fourth level you must have the confidence that your feelings are reasonable reactions to your client's behavior. Students generally lack this confidence and assume that their feelings are the result either of their own personal idiosyncrasies or of their incompetence as therapists. This has always been one of the most difficult aspects of training psychotherapy students. In addition to gaining more therapy experience yourself, observing other experienced therapists allows you the opportunity to check your emotional reactions against theirs. As you develop greater confidence in your personal reactions to your clients' behaviors, these will become an increasingly valuable source of information.

We have discussed only some of the complexities you will need to master in the course of your development as an accomplished clinician. We do not want to imply, however, that the more complex response is necessarily the better one. All levels of analysis can be used effectively, depending on the situation, the client, the goals of therapy, and your therapeutic orientation. You will find that different schools of therapy will focus on different levels. Our goal for beginners is that they gradually increase their comfort and effectiveness with each level. In this way they will have a wide range of tools to apply to a variety of situations.

The therapeutic alliance

As a final note in this chapter we wish to discuss the relationship between you and the client from a somewhat different perspective. This discussion should definitely not be considered a complete statement on the therapeutic relationship. Many volumes have been devoted to this topic alone. However, beginners have some common difficulties in forming their first relationships with clients that warrant being mentioned here.

A problem we've often encountered with student therapists is that they want to form a warm, supportive relationship with all clients. This is the stereotype of the "helpful therapeutic relationship," and initially it is a comfortable stance for students to adopt. However, not all clients respond well to this approach. Although we believe that a therapist must convey an attitude of concern and acceptance to all clients, this may take a variety of forms. Students have a difficult time realizing that a therapist can be concerned and accepting but at the same time be ready to confront the client.

The important point to keep in mind is that no single approach or stance will be appropriate to all clients. You may need direct confrontation and challenge with clients who are resistant to change or unwilling to recognize their own contributions to their problems. With others you may need to adopt a formal, distant stance in order to reduce the threat of the intimacy of a therapy relationship. The nature of the alliance you form with each client must be individually tailored for that person and their particular current situation. Your success in relating effectively to the widest range of clients will rest on your flexibility and breadth of skills in this area.

The qualities that lead you to determine what type of relationship is going to be most beneficial for any one client are very difficult to specify and really are beyond the scope of this book. Some examples might be illustrative.

A female client initially entered therapy saying that she had sexual difficulties. She did not feel comfortable discussing her sexual problems with anyone and was unsure whether anyone could help her. During the initial therapy session she repeatedly challenged the therapist and inquired about her qualifications and personal life. The therapist did not challenge her criticisms to any great extent; rather she attempted to communicate an acceptance of this woman's ambivalence toward therapy. The woman maintained a hostile and guarded attitude, but her desire to remain in therapy and to make efforts to deal directly with her sexual problems seemed to be increased by the therapist's attitude. It was clear over time that had the therapist responded to this client's challenging behavior with a parallel attitude, this woman would have either dropped out of therapy or used the therapeutic setting as an arena for combat.

Another example:

A couple entered therapy for marital difficulties. They were seen by a male and female cotherapy team in an effort to train them in some methods of communication. Very little progress was made. The wife consistently presented herself as making an effort to change, though frustrated by her husband's lack of involvement. After four or five sessions in this format, the female therapist requested a meeting with the wife alone. During this session the wife again presented herself in a rather dependent, victimized role. The female therapist responded, however, with a very direct confrontation. She challenged the client's statement that she had been trying to change and that her husband had not. Over a period of three or four additional meetings the therapist established a relationship with this woman which was far from warm and supportive, but rather was very challenging. She presented the client with a direct view of how she was coming across, which ultimately resulted in the client's recognizing how her behavior was contributing to the marital problems.

Another difficult aspect of the relationship between therapist and client is accepting that the therapy process is not always pleasant and that each session will not necessarily end on a good note. As stated previously, during the intake process you should create an atmosphere in which your client will want to confide in you and to come back for more sessions. At this stage you are careful to avoid ending a session on a disturbing note. However, as therapy progresses it may periodically be necessary to end an hour with some obviously bad feelings on the part of your client or yourself. This does not necessarily mean that the session has gone badly. The greatest amount of change may occur after such a session. As a beginning therapist you may feel very uncomfortable if your client leaves your office upset. Students often want to resolve the problem or make some effort to console the client.

Such efforts on your part can be detrimental. Again, this is an area in which increased experience, help from supervisors, and growing confidence in your own judgment can help you to make an appropriate decision.

We have discussed the therapeutic alliance thus far from the point of view of providing the most beneficial relationship for the client. It may be difficult for you to imagine yourself relating to a client in a manner that is atypical for you. It is important to recognize that your natural personal style of dealing with people will affect how you adapt to any type of relationship. It is often hard for students, who generally see themselves as supportive, understanding people, to relate to a client in a formal or challenging manner. To take such a stance may well feel awkward at first. You will find through experience that each role is interpreted in a slightly different manner by each therapist. The crucial factor in this learning experience is that you be flexible and willing to try a new way of relating.

In this chapter we have discussed some of the more subtle and complex aspects of the therapeutic interaction. You may find our suggestions difficult to implement at first, but it is hoped that they will become increasingly meaningful as you gain experience as a therapist. Developing more sophisticated skills will help you gain as much useful information as possible and take advantage of a wide spectrum of interventions. Many are subtle, require considerable experience, and are perfected only after lengthy clinical practice.

10

The client in crisis

There is a good chance that at some time during your training one of your clients will experience a life-threatening crisis. This is a difficult and frightening situation for any therapist. It is especially disturbing for beginners, who may be unsure of their skills and fearful of the consequences of their decisions.

When your client is in crisis it is often a time of crisis for you as a therapist. To some extent you will experience many of the feelings that the client has – anxiety, confusion, and uncertainty. These reactions are natural and understandable, but you must be in control of them when talking to your client. It is important to act calmly and rationally even though you may be worried and anxious. It is not helpful to your client if you panic. You should strive to convey an attitude of concern, but not alarm, and to model a rational problem-solving approach to the situation.

If this all sounds difficult to manage successfully, keep in mind that you do not have to handle an emergency situation entirely on your own. Students sometimes mistakenly see a client's crisis situation as a therapeutic failure and are reluctant to contact their supervisors for help. Do not hesitate to contact your supervisor immediately in a crisis situation. Emergencies are handled best when supervisory support is used liberally. It is also extremely helpful if you have anticipated the possibility of a crisis occurring and the options available to you ahead of time.

In this chapter we will discuss a general therapeutic strategy for handling emergencies. However, we will limit ourselves to discussing emergency situations during ongoing contact with a client. These will differ somewhat from crisis counseling, where you are called on to respond to an emergency with an unfamiliar client.

Crises: what to expect

It is important to keep in mind that the defining characteristic of a crisis is not the instigating event, but rather the client's inability to cope with a situation. An event that one client will take in stride will make another completely distraught and confused. Crises are usually caused by a catastrophic situation such as the death of a family member, a divorce, or the loss of a job. However, a series of apparently much more benign events may also precipitate a crisis. Again, you must judge the severity of the crisis by the client's reactions and not by the apparent seriousness of the instigating event.

As a general rule, you should expect a client in crisis to be upset, to be at least somewhat confused, and to display impaired judgment. Most clients will be anxious, although the degree of anxiety will vary widely. One client may be so overwhelmed with anxiety as to be in a disorganized state of panic. Another may be depressed, withdrawn, and uncommunicative. Clients in crisis are likely to have difficulty in making even very simple decisions, and they may want and need considerable direction from you. Feelings of dependency and helplessness may make some people ashamed to admit their difficulties, which will make your persistence in information gathering very important.

Although we have so far described some of the general responses you can expect from people in crisis, remember that each person will respond somewhat differently. One client may belligerently demand help from you, whereas another may want to terminate therapy. The specific reaction in each client will be filtered through and molded by the situation and his or her way of reacting to stress.

A general strategy for handling emergencies

Assisting clients in controlling their emotions. Helping your client calm down might be your initial focus of attention if he or she is too upset to communicate, reason, or listen effectively. A client may initially come to a session so anxious or angry as to have difficulty talking or else talking so rapidly as to be incomprehensible. One approach for slowing down your client is to tell him or her to stop for a moment, relax, and then resume talking. If the client continues talking very rapidly, it may help to modulate your own rate of speaking from its normal level to a much slower pace.

Your client may also find it calming simply to be able to talk at length about his or her problems. It is then often easier to sort out what has happened and to begin dealing with the problem in a rational manner.

Evaluating the severity of the risk. When faced with a client in crisis, your first priority should be to make a thorough assessment of the severity of the risk. You will have to judge whether your client is a danger to himself or herself or to others. People in such danger may require immediate hospitalization or some other preventive action on your part.

To make this evaluation you should deliberately and calmly explore what the client is feeling, thinking, and planning about all aspects of the crisis situation. Beginners have difficulty resisting the impulse to be helpful or to attempt to do something to relieve the tension prematurely – the client's *and* their own. This can have very unfortunate consequences. It may cut off the client's natural and useful expression of feeling and may stop the flow of valuable therapeutic information.

127

The simplest way to find out what your client has done or is planning to do is to ask directly. Usually the client's response is a good guide to future actions. (Although suicidal clients will sometimes deny self-destructive intentions, their behavior and affect are usually revealing.) Beginning therapists are often hesitant to ask their clients about the possibility of suicide because they are afraid they will give their clients ideas. This is an unrealistic notion that is not borne out by increased experience with clients.

You should learn whether your client believes there are people he or she can turn to during the time of crisis. A person in crisis needs to have people available who can be relied on to provide support and assistance. A person in crisis also needs to believe that he or she has available options. If your client thinks there is no way out or nothing left to do, it is a very dangerous sign. This increases the risk and clearly points to the necessity of working with the client immediately to develop some acceptable alternatives.

In assessing the situation, it is important to weigh the present crisis and the client's reactions to it against his or her history of undergoing and handling emergencies. This requires that you find out about the client's previous experience with situations in which he or she has felt unable to cope. You might ask such questions as, "Have you ever felt this way before?" "How often have you felt like this?" "What has caused you to feel this way before?" and, "What did you do then?" If you have weathered previous crises with a client, you can draw on the actions that proved successful earlier.

This information will be invaluable to you in making your decisions about how to proceed. Knowledge of how the client has reacted to similar situations in the past is another excellent predictor of how he or she will react now. For instance, if your client has acted impulsively in the past when faced with anxiety-producing situations, there is a good chance he or she may again act hastily in a poorly thought-out manner. Similarly, if your client has a history of responding in a dramatic and emotional way to situations in general, it may be expected that his or her reactions in emergency situations may have overblown qualities.

In making your assessment of how your client will respond, however, you cannot rely solely on your knowledge of previous behavior. You will have to take into consideration what is unique about the present situation. For instance, if your client's only friend moves away, his or her behavior may be very different from what it was in previous crises, and the risk of self-destructive acts may be higher. If your client has never before experienced a serious life crisis, you should remember that he or she will be more vulnerable to stress and may act uncharacteristically.

How you go about making your assessment of the gravity of the situation also depends on your therapeutic relationship with the client. For instance, you may have to ask many more questions of a new client than one you know well, because you probably already have knowledge of his or her strengths, weaknesses, potential resources, and likely ways of behaving. The support provided in your ongoing therapeutic relationship will also reduce the risk of your client acting impulsively or out of despair.

Thus far we have discussed crisis situations as if they were of singular character and type, which is not the case. Some crises are handled quickly, and others take considerable time to resolve. Although most clients experience crises infrequently, some are in constant turmoil. Usually you are contacted in an emergency situation because the client considers you to be a useful source of support. Some clients, however, may have other reasons. For instance, your client may call because he or she wants attention, is angry with you, or needs reassurance. While therapists are often concerned about inadvertently rewarding clients for attention-getting or manipulative behavior, as a general rule we believe that beginners should act conservatively and initially take at face value all potentially dangerous emergency situations. Only later, and after consultation with your supervisor, should a different approach be considered.

Helping the client clarify and focus on the problems. In order to cope with a crisis the client needs to gain a realistic perspective on what has happened and how this relates to his or her emotional state. Your client may be experiencing new emotions or a greater intensity of feeling than he or she has ever known before, and may find this confusing and frightening. Clarifying feelings and relating them to the specific causative issues can make the crisis seem less overwhelming. Some clients can develop this perspective by just talking about what has happened; others, however, may require your actively interpreting the situation for them. For example:

> A twenty-three-year-old woman was being seen in therapy for depression and difficulties in relating to men. She had temporarily been laid off from her job, and she called her therapist in a state of panic. She talked about financial worries and her inability to manage without a job. However, as the therapist sought clarification he discovered it was only a temporary layoff and the client had enough savings to meet expected expenses. After questioning her further, it seemed that she was primarily upset because she would miss the social life at work – her primary social outlet. The therapist expressed this hypothesis to the client, and she agreed that it made sense. Once the source of distress was clarified, she became much calmer. She and the therapist then began to develop a relevant plan for addressing these social concerns.

If a client is afraid that he or she will be incapable of coping with a crisis, you can compare the present situation with similar ones that the client has already experienced. This may remind the client that he or she has survived similar circumstances; furthermore, previously effective ways of coping may serve as a model for dealing with the present problems.

Other clients may need you to point out how their reactions are exacerbating the problem or preventing a constructive problem-solving response. For example:

> A forty-five-year-old man who had been seen in marital counseling lost his job during therapy. He scheduled a therapy session in a panic. He was afraid that he was too old to be hired again and would never find another job; that he could not afford to keep up the payments on the house or the car, which would soon be repossessed; and that everyone would think he was a failure.

The therapist pointed out the exaggerations in what the client was saying and how he was anticipating events that would probably not happen. These unfounded worries not only were further upsetting the client but were also keeping him from focusing on the immediate demands of the situation, such as beginning to look for a new job and adjusting family expenses.

Developing alternatives. Providing structure and focusing on the realistic problematic elements of the crisis can make it seem more manageable to a client. It is then easier to begin establishing new ways of coping. Clients in crisis often feel hopeless because they see no alternatives open to them, or the options they can think of are limited, unattractive, potentially harmful, or self-defeating. Your role in this situation is to help derive more constructive ways of responding.

Sometimes an appropriate course of action emerges from your conversation with the client, and he or she independently makes a decision or initiates a plan. For instance, your client may have had a fight with his or her spouse that ended with an agreement to seek a divorce. In the course of discussing the situation, your client decides to spend the night with a close friend and to call the spouse in the morning to talk in a less emotional atmosphere.

At other times your client may have difficulty making any decision or initiating any constructive action. In

131

these cases you must decide whether it is appropriate to intervene. This involves weighing the severity of the crisis against the dangers of taking over. Excessive or inappropriate intervention can result in the client's rebellion, unwanted fostering of dependency and helplessness, increase in the client's sense of incompetence, and damage to his or her self-esteem (which has already suffered because of the difficulties he or she is having in coping with the crisis). Because of these consequences it is generally important to allow the client to be as responsible as possible for the decisions and plans that need to be made.

However, in some emergency situations the "rules" of therapy are suspended. You may have to take some unorthodox action, for instance, personally making arrangements for an adolescent client to stay at a foster home. However, you should become involved to this extent only in exceptional cases, where it is clearly demanded by the risks to the people involved.

Very often you or your client will develop fairly specific plans. The actions may be as simple as acquiring or prescribing medication (the most frequently needed and used alternative), contacting a social agency, calling the police, or finding a friend to stay with a child. At other times a more complex course of action is called for, such as planning how to find a job. However, it is very important to keep in mind that deriving alternatives for a client does not necessarily mean that you have to come up with a solution. Many problems do not lend themselves to easy answers. What can be offered is a calm, rational, step-by-step problem-solving approach devoted to developing better plans for coping with a problem. For example:

> A client whose marriage ended after twenty-five years became despondent because she was lonely, wanted to remarry, but was not meeting eligible men. Although it was impossible to develop a simple course of action to find her a husband, the therapist promised to devote sessions to planning ways for her to meet men and to deal with her fears about being alone. Group therapy, a new treatment

approach, was also suggested to assist the client in dealing with her social anxieties.

Most of the time, merely mentioning alternatives is insufficient to help a client. You have to use your therapeutic skill to make them viable possibilities. Unfortunately, we can provide no neat prescription that can tell you how to do this. For example, clients may be hesitant initially to accept medication because of fears of becoming dependent on drugs. For medication to be a viable alternative you may have to discuss the clients' concerns and allay their fears in some way. This is often a complex therapeutic task requiring several sessions.

Agreeing on a course of action. It is important that you do not end your contact with a client until some reasonable decisions have been made and a concrete course of action has been agreed on. For example:

> Okay. We have agreed that you will stay with your parents tonight and call me when you arrive. I will call you there in an hour if I have not heard from you. I expect to see you again here tomorrow at nine.

> You will take your husband to the emergency room of the hospital, and I will meet you there.

It is also important in planning a course of action to build in contingencies for different outcomes. For example:

> If you can't reach me and you have to talk to someone, be sure to call the crisis hotline. Do you know the number?

> If your husband won't give you money to pay for groceries, then you will have to ask your parents for a loan.

Some clients will apparently agree with a course of action you have jointly established, although they are not really committed to the plan or can be easily dissuaded once they are no longer with you. Therefore you want to *emphasize your understanding* that they are agreeing with the plan and that this is an implicit contract between the two of you. You might say, for example:

133

You are promising me that you will call if you begin to feel suicidal.

You've agreed to call your parents, and I'm assuming you're going to follow through. Is there any reason why I shouldn't expect you to do it?

We both understand that we have an agreement that if you start feeling like you want a drink, you will call me or the crisis clinic, right?

Before allowing the client to leave, you should *summarize* the planned course of action your client is to take; for instance, "You have decided to leave your daughter with your parents for the next few weeks, and you will call the welfare department tomorrow about arranging for food stamps." You will want to maintain frequent contact with your client to find out whether he or she took any action, whether the action was effective, and whether the crisis is abating. Usually the crisis will pass, but if it does not, you should be aware of it and be available to intervene if necessary.

Our intention in this section is to give you a sense of how to develop alternatives with your client, and the examples should not be considered verbatim statements to make. The specific approach for each client cannot be prescribed ahead of time. As usual, you must be responsive to the unique characteristics of the crisis and the personality of the client to define your approach. Your own personal history in relating successfully and persuasively with a client is also an important consideration.

Providing support. Your behavior toward the client throughout the period of crisis is generally characterized by increased and consistent support and reassurance that you are available to help. You should particularly emphasize your availability to clients who have no other resources besides therapy on which to depend. Increasing your support often involves increasing your contact with the client. The frequency of contact is usually proportional to the severity of the crisis and the client's lack of family or friends to rely on.

In very serious situations you may give the client your home phone number with the instruction to call if needed. This is done only in rare and dangerous instances because of the problem of the client becoming overly dependent on you rather than relying on the resources in his or her daily environment.

A person in crisis may not perceive the importance of maintaining structure in his or her life and contact with other people. You may have to use your influence to ensure that the client uses the support available. For example, you may suggest that some arrangement be made so that the client is not completely alone, such as staying with a friend or a relative for a short period of time. Some clients will be quite difficult to convince, particularly those who are depressed and withdrawn and most in need of human contact. Again, in some rare and serious situations you may need to step in directly and enlist the help of the client's family and friends to make sure that the client is not alone.

Another potential support for clients in severe exceptional cases is hospitalization. You should consider this alternative when your client is behaving in bizarre or unpredictable ways, is unable to care for himself or herself, or is potentially dangerous. When the client is frightened by his or her experiences or impulses, it may be relatively easy to secure agreement to a voluntary hospital stay. However, hospitalization is often seen as a frightening or demoralizing alternative, and it may have a destructive impact on your treatment relationship. You must be able to portray it as an opportunity to gather resources together, and to utilize the medical and personal attention afforded by a full-time staff. A situation such as this tests both your therapeutic skills and your relationship with the client and should never be attempted without full supervisory support.

Using the crisis to therapeutic advantage. Thus far we have focused on the dangers and emotional distress of a crisis. There is another dimension to many crises: the potential for rapid and significant changes in the client's life. Crises often are times of decision and change. The uncertainty of the situation contributes to the client's subjective anxiety, but he or she may also be forced to take actions that would ordinarily be very difficult. For example:

> A twenty-nine-year-old married woman was being seen in therapy for depression. She was dissatisfied with her marriage, felt that her husband neglected her and that they were generally incompatible. She was very unsure of how to remedy the situation. For months she agonized over whether to stay married. She was afraid of being alone, unsure of her ability to manage by herself, and felt that she still might love her husband. One day she discovered that her husband was having an affair. This resulted in a major fight with her husband. She felt hurt and betrayed, and was very angry. She decided after the argument to separate from her husband, and within a week had found herself an apartment and had applied for a number of jobs.

A crisis period is also often a time when things come to a head and action is demanded on therapeutic issues. For instance, if a client has chronic problems because of excessive drinking, it may only be after an arrest for drunk driving and forfeiture of his or her license that the client will begin an alcohol treatment program. Similarly, it may only be after a child has run away from home that a recalcitrant parent will decide to enter family therapy. A crisis may jar some clients out of their usual perspective and allow them to see their behavior and the behavior of others in a new light. In this way the crisis may emphasize some issues you have been working on in therapy. For example:

> A couple was being seen at the wife's initiative in marriage counseling because of constant fighting. The hus-

band insisted that he could not understand why his wife was dissatisfied. The therapist had been attempting to make the husband understand how he was denying the validity of the wife's complaints and not accepting his own responsibilities for the problems in the marriage. It was only after the wife began a trial separation that the husband realized the severity of his wife's dissatisfaction and began to consider how he had been contributing to the problems.

Not only may your client see situations differently as a result of the crisis, but he or she may act in uncharacteristic ways. When normal rules of conduct and expectations are broken, your client may reveal new aspects of his or her personality. This may both contribute to a change in self-concept and reinforce some of your therapeutic aims.

A special case: handling the suicidal client

Being faced with a suicidal client is probably the most frightening emergency situation for any therapist. Suddenly you are faced with the reality that your client may kill himself or herself. You become overwhelmingly aware of how much your margin of error is narrowed and how crucial each response is. It is a common enough and distressing enough situation for beginners to warrant special discussion in this chapter.

An initial word of caution: You should always treat any statement of suicidal intent seriously. Never assume your client doesn't mean it. Only after investigating the issue thoroughly, and often after consultation with your supervisor, can you judge the severity of the situation.

Assessment. With a depressed client, it is always important to be on the alert for clues that indicate suicidal ideas or plans. For instance, if a seriously depressed client tells you there is nothing left to talk about, begins to thank you for all the help that you have provided, or tells you that you did all that could be done – think of *suicide* and inquire about it. Similarly, if your client begins to "place his life in order" (e.g., clean up closets, mail off all bills, do chores or assignments that are long overdue), recognize that these are danger signals that should be investigated.

Timing is also an important consideration in suicide. Very often the greatest risk of suicide is not when clients are in the absolute depths of a depression. At this time they may literally not have the energy to follow through on a plan of action. The greatest risk of suicide comes when clients begin to feel somewhat better and become more energetic. It is therefore very important to monitor your clients when they start improving and to maintain maximum attention and effort throughout this period. It is easy for a therapist to let up slightly as a client begins to improve. The therapist may feel personally exhausted or falsely optimistic and may mistakenly be less vigilant and supportive.

You can best assess the possibility of suicide by directly asking your client about it in a calm and straightforward manner. You might ask such questions as, "Are you thinking about killing [harming] yourself?" "Have you thought about this before?" "Have you thought about how you would do it?" "Have you done anything to carry out your plan?" and "What do you think are the chances of your killing [harming] yourself?" Often the client's statements about his or her intentions are a good predictor of future actions. Questions similar to those given help clarify the seriousness of the client's intentions to take some self-destructive action. Many clients will openly tell you about their suicidal feelings; however, others will not disclose them even when directly questioned. If your client denies any suicidal intentions but you are unconvinced because of other indications, you should take the same precautionary actions.

Do not feel required to make all the judgments and decisions about a potentially suicidal client by yourself.

In fact, most often it is advisable to acquire a second opinion. This assistance can be provided by your supervisor or another member of the supervisory staff. The timing of this consultation is important. It should occur after the client has talked to you at some length and you have an understanding of the situation and have developed some rapport. At an appropriate time and in a tactful way you can explain to the client your concerns and your desire to consult with another professional. Most clients will accept the need for consultation as a matter of course; it is the therapist, particularly a beginner, who becomes disturbed about having to turn to someone else for assistance. It is important that you present it in a composed, matter-of-fact way so that the client does not view your seeking help from a colleague as a rejection or as panic on your part.

Therapeutic response. Your general therapeutic approach to a suicidal client will not differ from your response to other serious emergency situations. However, you will be more likely to intervene forcefully and to push your therapeutic prerogatives to their limits.

In providing therapeutic assistance to a suicidal client it is necessary to provide support and quickly develop more constructive alternatives. Often the most valuable assistance you can provide to your client is your own accessibility. To assure your availability you may want to give your client your home phone number with instructions to call if he or she is feeling despondent. Frequent scheduling of sessions, possibly even daily, provides an important future commitment. A client may not kill himself or herself today because of an appointment to see you tomorrow. On the other hand, it is a dangerous sign if your client cancels a scheduled appointment. You should not let this go by without contacting him or her to make some type of further arrangement.

In addition to the support you provide, it will usually be necessary to marshall the help of available friends and family during a crisis. For instance, if it is at all possible, a suicidal individual should not be left alone. You will need to work with your client in making these arrangements. Unfortunately, severely depressed persons very often do not want to be around other people. Once they are with someone else their feelings about this often change, but initially you may have to use your influence or authority to convince them. For instance, you might state that it is your professional opinion that the client must stay with someone for the next week. To another client you might present a forced-choice option, that is, he or she will either stay with a friend for the next week or enter the hospital.

Although the use of appropriate medication is also often vitally necessary with suicidal clients, the dosage must be carefully monitored. To ensure that the client follows through you might want to make the appointment or even accompany him or her to the doctor's office.

Your therapeutic aim in treating a suicidal client is to get your client through the suicidal impulse period, which may be relatively short. A basic rule is to do anything that works, that allows the client to pass through the highest risk period safely. The approach and available alternatives vary with each client. These may be very unorthodox actions which you would never use in ordinary therapy. For instance, you might appeal to the client's religious beliefs or to his or her family obligations if this will forestall a suicidal act.

As a word of warning, it is generally ineffective to try to talk the client out of his or her feelings or to provide empty reassurance. Such approaches as, "It's not that bad," and, "Everyone feels blue once in a while," which do not consider the client's feelings, probably alienate him or her more than anything else. Similarly, trying to reassure the client ("It will all work out," or, "Don't worry. She will come back") is also usually ineffective.

The decision to hospitalize a suicidal client is difficult to make, and you will want to discuss it at length with your supervisor. Obviously, hospitalization must be considered when there is a serious possibility that a client may kill himself or herself. However, as stated previously, many clients will not want to be hospitalized, even though they are seriously suicidal. You will have to weigh the clients' opposition and the infringement of freedom that they will tolerate against the advantages of a hospital stay (e.g., availability of medical attention, constant supervision, and the opportunity to get away from a stressful environment). If you believe hospitalization is the best plan, you may have to use all your power and influence as a therapist to persuade your client.

To have someone hospitalized against his or her will is often difficult and may cause irreparable damage to your treatment relationship. Its feasibility also varies depending on the legal codes in your state. You should know what the legal requirements are so that you are prepared to initiate commitment procedures if the need arises. At the present time there is a general trend to allow hospitalization of persons against their will only if it can be *proved* that they are a danger to themselves or others.

A final note

After having dealt with a client in crisis, most beginning therapists are concerned about having responded appropriately. Did they do the right thing, and did they do enough? These are questions you cannot answer by yourself. Your supervisor can provide you with the most useful feedback. However, it is important for you not to confuse an appropriate response with a successful outcome. It is not always possible to solve a client's problems, alleviate his or her distress, or even stop a suicide. If a person is intent on suicide he or she may succeed even on a security ward. This does not mean that you should do less than your maximum effort, but your maximum effort is all that is possible.

11
Termination

Beginning therapists expect that therapy will end smoothly at some ideal time when the client is relieved of all problems and has learned to master new difficulties as they arise. Unfortunately, this rarely happens. The ending of therapy usually represents a compromise between hoped-for changes and limitations arising from waning motivation, the subjective discomfort of being in therapy, its cost, and a variety of other factors.

Handling termination is typically difficult for students. They find themselves caught off guard by a client's announcing the decision to terminate; they too eagerly decide to terminate when the client begins to feel better; or they continue seeing a client long after it is productive because they don't know how or when to make the decision to end. Beginners make their first mistake by not considering the issue of ending therapy at the start. Termination is integrally related to the goals of treatment and can only be considered within this context. Therefore when you are formulating treatment objectives, it is wise to give some thought to the criteria you might use to determine when these goals have been met.

In this chapter we will be presenting some guidelines for making the decision to terminate therapy and some practical advice on how to implement this decision. We will also provide guidance about what to do when a client wants to terminate unexpectedly. The chapter will conclude with a discussion of how these ideas apply when a client is transferred to another therapist.

How to terminate a client

Making the decision to bring up the issue. When you begin to consider the idea of terminating a client, your first task is to determine your reasons for ending therapy at this particular time. We strongly recommend you explore the topic in depth with your supervisor. Outside objectivity is often critically important because it is tempting to decide to quit for personal reasons – for instance, because you don't know what else to do or don't feel competent to help the client. Being aware of your personal feelings while avoiding basing the decision on them is a difficult task, one with which a supervisor may be very helpful.

It is generally appropriate to bring up the question of termination with a client when you believe either that the client has reached his or her therapy goals or that further progress is not possible at this time. Articulating the objectives of therapy and assessing its progress will be fairly straightforward in some cases, yet very elusive in others. For example, in treatment for sexual dysfunction the desired outcome is usually clear, and progress can be fairly easily measured. However, other clients consult you about vague problems. Therapeutic goals are more difficult to define and progress more difficult to measure, for example, when the client complains of diffuse dissatisfaction with relationships or general apathy. Remember, however, that perfection in achievement of goals is not required and rarely occurs. A reasonable approximation is usually acceptable.

The client's rate of progress in reaching treatment goals is also an important matter to consider in making any decision about discontinuing therapy. If the treatment is no longer significantly helping a client change or feel better, its usefulness should be questioned. Even if a client is making exceedingly slow yet visible progress, he or she may profit from a break from therapy, with the option of reentering later. Careful consideration is always

143

in order, because slow and arduous progress is sometimes followed by significant breakthroughs.

At times you may suspect that continued therapy will not result in significant progress because the client lacks the motivation to change. As we will discuss more fully later in the chapter, clients have many reasons for seeking therapy; some do not involve a desire for change or personal development. You will encounter clients who want to remain in therapy because they are afraid of having to cope with future problems on their own; others are in treatment to have someone else make their decisions or even to avoid making changes. There will be times when a client is motivated to change but is hampered by his or her marital, financial, or job situation. All these factors affect the advisability of continuing.

Decisions about discontinuing therapy weigh the time, effort, and cost of therapy against its expected gains for the client. They are complicated judgments for a beginner, and you will probably need the assistance of your supervisor to consider them adequately.

How to discuss termination with a client. Your usual first step is to describe in detail your reasons for considering termination. Usually this is explained within the context of the goals of therapy and the changes and achievements, or lack of them, that have occurred over the course of treatment.

At first glance this appears to be a fairly straightforward task. However, it can be exceedingly difficult to carry out effectively, particularly if the client has not anticipated it or objects to the idea. Beginning students are often reluctant to initiate the topic of termination because they are concerned about the client's possible negative reactions – and with good reason. It is critical to explore thoroughly the client's thoughts and feelings in reaction to your suggestion. Although it varies with each client and within each therapeutic relationship, clients commonly perceive termination as a failure. They may feel rejected or abandoned by the therapist. It is generally a good idea to explore the possibility of these reactions, even though your client may not spontaneously mention them.

Both you and the client should have ample opportunity to exchange opinions about and reactions to the reasons for terminating that you have suggested. Some clients will react with relief because they have run out of things to bring up but don't want to hurt your feelings by leaving therapy. Others will feel devastated and abandoned and will react with a dramatic increase in problem behaviors. We cannot delineate each possible reaction; however, we suggest that you give some thought to your client's possible reactions *before* bringing up the issue so that you will be prepared for what may happen.

Initiating a discussion of termination does not necessarily mean that therapy has to end. Your client may disagree with you and bring up a pressing concern that may change your mind. The impact of bringing up termination and the subsequent discussion may have a marked and beneficial effect on the continuing course of therapy. For instance, it is possible that the exchange will instigate changes in a recalcitrant client's behavior and attitudes toward therapy. This can allow progress to resume or even begin for the first time. On the other hand, you may discover that the client has been dissatisfied with therapy but has been unwilling to bring it up. The discussion may clarify issues for both of you and may lead to significant changes in the course of therapy. For example:

A couple being seen for orgasmic dysfunction continually failed to carry out homework assignments and blamed their lack of progress on the student therapists' incompetence. After six weeks of attempting to make the requested changes in the treatment format with little success, the therapists confronted the couple with their lack of motivation, resistance, and intellectual defensiveness and proposed the possibility of termination. For the first time the clients considered this alternative to explain their

145

lack of progress and renegotiated with the therapists to continue therapy for a specified number of sessions to assess whether any change could be made.

Perhaps the most difficult situation for any therapist, novice or expert, is the case where the client insists on continuing treatment even though you feel that no progress is being made or that therapy is destructive to the client's growth, independence, or problem-solving abilities. The subtleties of these types of cases require extensive consultation with your supervisor, and you must allow adequate time to explore them thoroughly with the client. At some point you may have to be prepared to end therapy even though the client strenuously objects to it and feels personally rejected by you. This situation tests even the most competent therapist and causes beginners to agonize about the accuracy of their judgments.

Ending therapy and providing closure. You should not terminate therapy abruptly, particularly if you have had a long-standing relationship with the client. Often it is helpful to allow a period of time (perhaps two to four additional sessions) to work through the termination process and obtain closure. You may wish to meet with the client more infrequently for a time or build in trial periods of "independence" interspersed with the regular level of therapeutic contact. During the ending phases of therapy you will probably want to make fewer interventions, allow the client to make more decisions, and encourage him or her to take on greater responsibility for the sessions. You and the client are likely to spend more time planning for the future – anticipating problems and speculating on how the client might handle them. The tenor of the sessions sometimes changes, with the therapist being less formal and more self-disclosing. Often a major focus of this period is the client-therapist relationship and its imminent termination.

A general attitude of change and transition is introduced into the sessions. This occurs in many ways, some

146

subtle and some obvious, all of which, however, indicate the client's more independent, secure, and strengthened status. In this way you slowly remove your formal support and structure and approximate what it will be like for the client in the future without therapy.

During the last therapy sessions it is important to provide some closure on the experience for the client. This may be done by giving an overview of what has occurred in therapy and discussing with the client the changes that have been made. Remember to elicit the client's point of view of these topics as well as to offer your own, because the discrepancies may be large and may warrant extended discussion.

It is also important to keep in mind that termination does not imply that the changes initiated by therapy will not continue. The client may well continue to improve and grow as initial changes produce positive results in his or her life and self-perception. Finally, the option of entering therapy again should be presented as a viable and acceptable possibility for the future. You should mention this in such a way that it does not imply failure for the client if he or she decides that therapy would again be helpful.

What to do when your client suggests termination

There is a great deal of difference between the equivocal client who brings up the topic of ending therapy for discussion and the client who has already made the decision and presents it to you as a fait accompli. Many of your clients will terminate simply and finally by never returning to meet with you. Student therapists find this particularly frustrating and disappointing, but it is common and you must learn to accept it.

Some abrupt or premature terminations can be avoided by being alert to clues that the client is thinking about quitting and bringing it up for open discussion before the decision is final. Although the client may not openly state his or her intentions to quit treatment, various other remarks may be revealing; for example, "I don't have anything to talk about any more," "I don't think this therapy is helping," or, "I don't see how that is important to my problems." Frequent lateness or missed appointments are other indicators that a client is getting ready to quit.

We will devote most of this discussion to the situation in which you have some room to negotiate. When a client has already made a firm decision you are left with very few alternatives, particularly if he or she refuses to come in for one last session. At that time you and the client can bring some closure to the therapy experience, even though you may still not agree about the advisability of terminating.

Evaluating the client's reasons for terminating. When a client wants to terminate, your first response should be to listen and ask questions until you understand the reasons. Beginners need to keep in mind that wishing to terminate will not always be directly related to what has occurred in therapy sessions. It will most likely involve an interaction between (1) progress and goal attainment; (2) what is currently happening in the process of therapy itself; (3) the level of subjective discomfort; and (4) the client's financial, social, and work situation. Change in any one of these areas may shift the balance in the client's weighing of the costs and benefits of treatment and can trigger a desire to terminate.

As a general rule, clients want to quit therapy when they feel better. This may mean that the problem situation has been resolved to their satisfaction, that they have learned better coping skills, or simply that external events have changed to reduce their stresses. It is important to remember that therapists and clients frequently have divergent objectives for therapy. You are being trained to work toward certain types of changes in the client's behavior or personality. Yet this might not coincide with the client's goals. People seek out therapy because, among other things, they want advice, affirmation of their behavior, or a chance to ventilate their feelings.

Clients often expect less from therapy than you do. Some will want to end treatment just about the time you think you are getting started. On the other hand, sometimes the client recognizes his or her improvement and decreased need for therapy earlier, and more accurately, than the therapist. It may be appropriate for the client to terminate even though you perceive some areas worthy of further consideration. The client may benefit from being on his or her own, and the continuation of therapy may actually be a hindrance by encouraging dependence or fostering feelings of helplessness and inadequacy. Whatever the circumstance, the client has the final decision on termination, and this must be respected.

A client's statement of wanting to terminate therapy must not be taken at face value. An announcement that one is terminating is generally a good way to get the therapist's attention. It may also be a way for the client indirectly to tell you something that he or she is not willing to say directly – for example, that you have not been involved, supportive, or attentive enough lately. When a client is angry or hurt it may be easier to say, "I quit," than to express the feelings openly. Similarly, clients may terminate to avoid feelings of anxiety or failure. Quitting may mask the client's feelings of having failed you by not following your suggestions; it may be a way of coping with frightening changes engendered by therapy.

As mentioned earlier, events outside of therapy also often contribute to a client's wish to terminate. The life circumstances that brought him or her to treatment may change; a troubled marriage may dissolve, a separation may become a reconciliation, or a difficult boss may be transferred. On the other hand, family and friends may apply pressure to the client to quit because they do not approve of the changes made, even though you see them as beneficial. For example:

A thirty-four-year-old married woman with four children entered therapy because she was severely depressed. Almost all her time was spent at home with either her children or her husband, who liked to stay at home after work and on weekends. In her interactions with her husband she was passive and generally did what her husband told her to do. As a result of therapy, the woman became more assertive with her husband and began spending considerably more time away from home, doing things with her friends. The woman became less depressed, but the husband became angry about how she was now behaving, and they began having major fights. The husband blamed therapy for the changes in his wife's behavior and demanded that she end therapy or he would leave her. The woman then ended therapy.

Another possible reason for termination may be changes in the client's financial situation. He or she may no longer be able to afford the fee but may be embarrassed to tell you. However, beware of accepting financial and other reasons outside of the therapeutic situation for terminating without thoroughly exploring the client's feelings and thoughts about treatment itself. Money is often used as an indirect way of terminating therapy for other reasons. It is often easier for clients to say they cannot afford therapy than directly to state their dissatisfaction with you or with treatment.

Exploring and evaluating a client's wish to terminate can be highly complicated. Your response should be similar to your response to other equally complicated treatment issues. You must explore the limits of the client's awareness as thoroughly as possible, although the client may not be able to tell you what you want to know. You must speculate about why the client is bringing up termination, and why now. This process requires you to consider all you know about the client and what has been going on inside and outside therapy. Then you will bring up your speculations with the client and, if possible, use them to further the client's learning and personal growth.

Handling your own feelings. You may have a wide variety of emotional reactions to a client who announces his or her intention to terminate. Reactions range from a sense of relief to feelings of sadness, anger, rejection, and anxiety. If the client presented a difficult set of problems for which you foresaw no easy solutions, you may feel relieved of the burden of treatment. Similarly, if a client was difficult to interact with, hostile, or boring, you may be secretly glad not to have to see him or her anymore. It may be tempting to allow such a client to terminate without discussing the issue thoroughly in an objective way. Other considerations, such as the size of your case load, your feelings toward your supervisor, or the stresses of your own personal life may also influence your feelings about a client terminating.

Beginners often get upset when a client wishes to terminate because they view it as either a therapeutic failure or a personal rejection. They deprecate their abilities as a therapist or become angry at the client for not behaving as they would like. Both reactions are personalized and inappropriate, but it is difficult for students to learn to be objective about these matters. Beginners also even mistakenly encourage clients to continue therapy out of the fear of being negatively evaluated by their supervisor if a client leaves. A large part of learning to be a good psychotherapist is learning to separate these personal feelings from your professional evaluation of the client's best interests. These things do not come either quickly or easily, however, and you may expect to struggle with them for some time.

What if you don't agree? It is not always possible to reach a mutually satisfactory agreement through your discussion and negotiations with the client. In the end it is the client's decision and solely under his or her control. Sometimes the client will leave against your advice, and you will have to accept that reality.

If you have a good working relationship you may be

able to negotiate a more mutually satisfactory termination point. For example, you might ask a client to continue for a certain number of sessions to complete the business of therapy. The option of a time-limited format is sometimes more acceptable to a client who wishes to leave than is an open-ended contract.

We believe that you should not strongly attempt to influence the decision if a client is determined to leave unless you believe it is a mistake that seriously threatens his or her functioning. When you believe the client is in jeopardy, you may have to use all your supervisory resources, your therapeutic abilities, and your relationship with the client to convince him or her to remain in therapy.

Transferring a client to another therapist

Transfer because of leaving your training setting. The requirements and restrictions inherent in training settings may call for transferring your clients to other therapists before their treatment goals are reached. The amount of time beginning therapists remain in one setting or institution is usually limited and known in advance. You should include these time limitations in your planning when the therapy goals are being formulated. The client ought to know about the possibility of referral long before the end of your contact so that he or she can be prepared for the change of therapists.

It is actually quite problematic to refer a client successfully to another therapist. In some cases, even though therapy is not complete, it may be better to terminate than to introduce a new therapist. Many clients are simply unwilling to make another personal investment of that magnitude, particularly if they have been very involved with you. Even though your contact is ending because of reasons beyond your control, a client may still have feelings of rejection and view transferral

152

as a reflection on him or her. Extended discussion, reassurance, and repeated urging are often required to complete a referral.

Even though your reasons for ending therapy with the client are different from those in termination, many of the issues and ways of concluding are similar. These guidelines are not repeated in detail here, because they are discussed earlier in the chapter. However, the general approach of exploration of the client's feelings, discussion and negotiation, and development of closure on the experience is still appropriate. As with termination, some planning or discussion of future problems should occur, with particular reference to the difficulties the client may anticipate in feeling comfortable with and learning to trust a new therapist.

Transfer for personal reasons. Sometimes lack of progress in therapy may be due to the specific interaction between you and your client. Your personality styles or value systems may conflict, or you may have difficulty remaining objective about the client's problems for personal reasons. If you think these types of complications are interfering with your ability to treat the client effectively, you may need to consider transferring him or her to another therapist. This is a very difficult judgment to make, and it is usually made in conjunction with the supervisor after a considerable period of time. However, it is valid to transfer a client for personal reasons, and this situation occurs with beginners and experienced therapists alike. Because this is a major move, it should not be implemented without careful consideration. Nothing is accomplished by transferring a difficult and unpleasant client to another therapist who will have the same difficulties.

It is more difficult for both the client and the therapist to make a transfer when personal reasons are involved. The situation often forces both the beginning therapist and his or her client to question themselves and their

153

abilities to relate to other people. Extensive supervisory consultation and support are required in order to cope with the personal questions you as the therapist may have and to handle the situation constructively and effectively with the client.

In summary, termination is an important aspect of the entire therapy process and requires considerable time and effort to be handled properly. It is a part of clinical work that all too often receives short shrift because of lack of planning and preparation. We hope to have given you some guidelines to consider throughout the course of treatment so that its ending will not come as a surprise.

12
Record keeping

Professional standards and institutional policies usually require therapists to make some written documentation of client contacts. Experienced professionals generally acknowledge the importance of keeping good records. However, a great discrepancy exists between these standards and what is actually done. Most therapists maintain some records, but these are often scribbled notes rather than up-to-date files.

We can empathize with students' reluctance to spend large amounts of time working on records. Clinicians are generally "people oriented" and find client contact more interesting and compelling than solitary report writing. Also, students tend to think they will remember everything that happened during a session with a client. Writing it all down is time-consuming, sometimes painful, and seems like wasted effort. Reports often go unnoticed by supervisors or administrative personnel. Students usually receive neither positive nor negative feedback about their record keeping, except when a required report has *not* been written. Unfortunately, the importance and value of keeping appropriate records often only become clear when the records are needed but not available. It is only then that students, or experienced therapists, begin in earnest to document fully what transpires during therapy.

Reasons for keeping records

Facilitation of treatment. Some of the purposes served by keeping good records may not be initially evident to you.

155

Your own treatment skills and your client's progress will be enhanced in a number of ways by record keeping. For example, it is useful before each session to review your notes briefly to remind yourself of important events and themes of prior sessions. Your notes should indicate pressing concerns left unresolved at the end of the last visit. The importance of this review is particularly obvious in behavioral therapies, which often require considerable detailed monitoring of the client's actions or emotions inside and outside therapy sessions. It is most embarrassing as well as destructive to the treatment process to request that your client do something between sessions and then forget to ask about it.

Your notes not only assist you in recollecting what transpired in previous sessions, but can also serve as reminders of therapeutic material or aspects of the treatment plan you wish to pursue in a future session. You may jot down a note indicating the need to clarify or examine some issue next session (e.g., to review some aspects of the client's history). At other times you may record an emotional reaction or some other aspect of the client's report that was of therapeutic interest but was not examined because it was of less immediate importance than the ongoing topic. You may also use your records as a way of reminding yourself about some plan of action you want to take in the future, for example, to ingore a certain topic the client uses to divert the conversation from more anxiety-provoking areas.

A great many things go on during most therapy sessions. It is easy to become so immersed in secondary issues and ongoing daily events that you lose sight of the major treatment goals. However, when you summarize a session in your reports, you are forced to develop some needed distance from each individual session and to consider the overall central therapeutic issues. This is especially necessary in therapy that deals with diffuse problems in an unstructured format, where the treatment goals may be somewhat abstract and remote.

The process of conceptualizing involved in report writing also helps you to examine regularly and consistently whether therapy is being helpful and what particular procedures are proving useful to your client. This issue of the client's progress is a critical one that is all too often neglected until the ending point of therapy arrives. Regular consideration of progress in your report writing can guide you in ongoing treatment evaluation and planning.

Record keeping for training purposes. During their training, students are often required to make a separate set of detailed notes for their supervisory meetings. The necessity for these notes varies, depending on the use and accessibility of audio or video recording equipment; however, taking detailed notes after a session is often a useful training device in that it forces you not only to remember what your client said, but also to observe and remember his or her actions and emotions during the session. The relationship of the client's affect and behavior to what is said during the session is a critical element of the therapeutic process. You will want to notice and record this complex picture for your own edification and training, and for discussion with your supervisor.

For example, it is worthwhile to note voice fluctuations, bodily movements and posture, the appearance of nervous mannerisms, and any changes in emotion. You will need to attend to what precipitated these events and the matters being discussed when these changes occurred. Similarly, you will want to consider how *your* actions during the sessions affected the client's behavior and emotions.

It takes considerable experience to learn to discern these complex relationships from the involved and often confusing events of a therapy session. You are initially not expected to note every subtle nuance and change occurring during therapy; however, careful and thoughtful note taking will help you develop this skill.

Administrative reasons. Record keeping also serves to document treatment for possible future reference. Your impressions of the client and the course of therapy can be invaluable to a wide variety of sources with whom your client will have contact in the future. Remember, however, that information about treatment is privileged and can normally be supplied *only* in response to a written request by the client. It is impossible to predict who might need the relevant information about your client. It might be another therapist or colleague, some social, governmental, or judicial agency, or even yourself some time in the future. Since you do not know who might need the records or for what purpose, they should be complete so that the relevant information can be selected. The unavailability of information on prior therapeutic contacts not only is personally frustrating to the other professional, but can impair the effectiveness and quality of treatment that your client receives in the future.

The information contained in your records is also vitally important if someone else has to treat your client when you are not available. Emergencies may arise for your client when you cannot be reached because of vacations, illnesses, or a variety of personal reasons. Another staff member will probably have to rely on your written records to provide the needed information about your therapeutic approach and any pressing issue that should be attended to.

If you are working in any setting where other professionals or students routinely have contact with your client or monitor your treatment, your records provide important, often vital information about the status of the client and the therapy approach that you are using. For example, your supervisor may wish to examine your records regularly in order to ensure that the client is receiving adequate treatment. In any event, your reports should be sufficiently complete and up to date that, if necessary, someone can examine them and find out what is happening with the case.

158

Legal reasons. Besides the therapeutic and administrative functions served by keeping records, your written records may be needed in case of litigation involving your client. Your records not only serve as reminders to you of the events of therapy, but also constitute formal documentation of what transpired, which will carry weight in legal proceedings. It is particularly important to describe fully any situations that may have legal implications or repercussions, such as an attempted suicide or homicide, a minor running away from home, a sexual advance made by your client, or major therapy decisions such as termination.

When documenting material that may be of legal significance, it is important that you describe the entire situation as fully as possible. You need to note the precipitating events, the client's behavior and emotional reactions, your response, and whatever resolution occurred. It is also necessary to describe any actions you have taken about the client's situation that occur outside the therapy session; for example, you may have requested an evaluation of suicide potential by an experienced therapist or discussed the situation with your supervisor. In your records be sure to include the consultant's opinions about the situation and the recommended actions to be taken.

Some thoughts to keep in mind when writing reports

When writing reports you will be faced with a conflict between conciseness and the necessity of providing enough information. We have discovered that many beginning therapists are initially too comprehensive. Much of this information may be needed in their notes for supervision (e.g., verbatim quotes or detailed accounts of the client's experience) but is not appropriate for the official records. However, with experience, beginning therapists learn what information is essential to include in their records and what information can be omitted. In the latter part of this chapter we will outline what to include in the various reports you will be called on to write. However, these are only general suggestions. You will have to use your best judgment in each particular case and be guided by any feedback you receive.

You can never know the final destination or reader of your records after they have been sent in response to your client's request. Your client may have contact with a wide variety of professional sources who are specifically interested in your records. Beyond these individuals, other professionals may receive your records if the client's file is later forwarded by this second party. In addition, you can never be sure how someone will use your records in the future. Your client may be questioned about something you have noted, or may even be given the report to read. Therefore you should be as precise as possible in your writing, aiming for minimum interpretive error on the reader's part. As a rule, you should attempt to be descriptive in your language and to label your opinions as such when you give them. For instance, it is important to be judicious in your choice of words and to avoid value-laden words, such as *promiscuous* or *unreliable,* which reflect your opinions. It is preferable to describe the events or behaviors in question rather than to use a label that may be misinterpreted.

A closely related dilemma involves whether you should include information in your records that is potentially damaging to your client, but is not essential to therapy. A client may disclose information that he or she has acted illegally, immorally, or indiscreetly, but these actions have no relevance or bearing on the client's present life or on therapeutic issues. An example of this situation would be a mental health professional you are seeing in therapy who tells you that at one time he or she had sexual relations with a client. This fact is irrelevant to your client's reasons for entering therapy, and if it became known to members of the professional community it would have detrimental consequences. What should you include in your records about this incident? As a general rule, we believe that you have a higher responsibility to protect your client from inadvertent exposure to damaging information than to have totally complete records. When you are faced with decisions about what to include in your written records, we believe a useful guide is whether the client would suffer *unnecessarily* if the records somehow come into the wrong hands.

You will be faced with a more difficult problem if your client discusses potentially damaging information that is related to therapy. Here you will have to use the standard policy at your institution and your individual judgment to guide your decisions about what to include and what to omit. Each situation like this will be different, and there are no simple rules to guide you. It is important to be flexible and to weigh the relative merits of your alternatives. For instance, if you are treating someone for compulsive shoplifting, this, of course, would have to be mentioned in your notes. On the other hand, it probably would not be necessary to include the times and places your client stole things.

Types of records

Good professional practice typically dictates that a client's record consist of an intake report, regular progress notes, and a termination summary. The specific format and types of report expected of beginning therapists will vary, depending on the requirements of each particular setting. A description of the specific types of report and the information to be included most likely has been made available to you. In this section we will briefly describe these reports and their usual formats; however, any instruction you receive at your training setting should serve as your specific guide for report writing.

Intake report. Your first report on a client is usually a written summary of the intake interview. The chapter on giving a staffing report presents a detailed description of the essential information usually included in your written report on the intake interview:

orienting information
presenting problem
current functioning
supporting history
testing and consultations
clinical judgments and diagnosis
treatment recommendations

In addition, a summary of the conclusions about diagnosis and treatment developed during the staffing conference is often incorporated into the final intake report, although sometimes it is presented separately.

The description of the treatment plan usually includes specification of the goals of therapy, some description of the procedures to be used and any risks involved, an estimate of the expected length of treatment, and the probability of successful outcome. This detailed statement of a treatment plan is a fairly recent development in the mental health field and reflects both changes in perspective by members within the field and growing regulation of professional practice by various agencies. A more clearly defined proposal for treatment enables clients (and any third party involved in payment) to make better decisions about the relevance and adequacy of the services offered. It also forces the clinician to consider responsibly the cost to the client versus the advantages to be gained.

When writing your intake report, care should be taken to present the information in an organized and coherent fashion. A verbatim repetition of your oral staffing report will probably come across as rambling when written. You should strive to be clear and succinct and to pare away any unnecessary commentary. If the information is presented in a lengthy and disorganized manner, people who might use your report will often not take the time to read it, and what you have learned about the client may be lost to them.

162

It should also be mentioned that the intake report may be useful to you during treatment. You may refer to your report if you are unclear about, or have forgotten, some important information. More importantly, your intake report provides you with a baseline against which you can measure progress toward treatment goals. By reviewing your intake report you may also be reminded of what were initially perceived as important therapeutic issues, which may have been inadvertently neglected in the course of treatment.

Progress notes. To document your treatment fully you will need to record all contacts with your client, including important telephone conversations as well as contact with other professionals or involved parties (e.g., spouses, parents, etc.). However, routinely your progress notes will consist of a brief description of the essential details of your regular sessions with a client. They should include enough information so that the reader (or you in the future) can follow the course of therapy session by session.

A typical progress note begins with a brief description of the client's appearance, emotional state, and how he or she behaved during the session. For example:

> The client seemed very tense and agitated during the session. She continually was shifting her position, wringing her hands, or fidgeting with her dress or belt.

> The client was fifteen minutes late for the session, his clothes were rumpled, and he had not shaved.

You should also summarize the pertinent information discussed and the issues raised during the sessions, including specification of any changes in the client's life situation or behavior. For example:

> The client reported that she was continuing to initiate contact with people and not staying at home waiting for others to call her when feeling lonely and depressed. She was somewhat discouraged because not all her efforts had succeeded. However, she was in a more optimistic

163

mood by the end of the session, after discussing her successful efforts and reviewing the issue of her perfectionistic standards.

It is also important that you indicate what actions you take (e.g., interpretations, suggestions, assignments). For example:

> The client reported that he had volunteered for yet another committee assignment at work. I pointed out this was the third committee he had volunteered for and suggested that this might be another way of avoiding being at home with his wife. He admitted that in fact he and his wife were frequently fighting and he wanted to avoid being at home. I suggested some new ways for him to express his disagreements with his wife and made an assignment for him to bring up at least one issue for discussion this week.

Finally, a summary of the course of therapy and the client's progress should be mentioned. For example:

> The client's depression is decreasing as she continues to initiate contact with people and she is becoming more assertive. She is also becoming increasingly more aware of how her perfectionism causes her to devalue herself.

Termination report. Similar to the intake report, the termination report is a major, fairly detailed statement; however, the emphasis of this report is primarily on describing what transpired during therapy and how it ended. Typically, your termination report begins with a brief statement summarizing the contact you have had with the client: when therapy began, the frequency of sessions, the regularity of contact, and the date therapy ended. For example:

> The client was seen for her intake interview on July 6, 1976, and was scheduled for weekly sessions beginning on July 13, 1976. She frequently did not come to appointments and was actually seen for only six sessions between the initial intake and the final session on October 12, 1976.

164

You should follow with a summary of the course of therapy, detailing the major events and changes that occurred. For example:

> The client's initial concerns centered around the difficulties he was experiencing in his marriage. He reported frequent fights and a general sense of dissatisfaction. The emphasis of discussion during the initial sessions was on identifying the sources of satisfaction and dissatisfaction in the marriage. This led to a later examination of how the client himself was contributing to the marital problems. The last few sessions involved a discussion of the priorities in the client's life. At the time of termination he decided that he did in fact want to resolve the difficulties in the marriage and believed marriage counseling was needed.

The issue of the client's progress and why you believe change did or did not occur needs to be addressed in a termination report. Mention should also be made of the client's attitude toward therapy, your opinion of his or her motivation to change, and your impression of the client's satisfaction or dissatisfaction with treatment.

The client's experiences with you – both positive and negative – will provide a "set" that can either facilitate or hinder future treatment contacts. Knowledge of the obstacles and sensitive areas of past treatment can help another therapist avoid the same pitfalls. For example:

> The client reported being under considerable subjective discomfort and seemed very motivated to alter his situation. Although moderately defensive, he would generally spontaneously disclose problem areas, give consideration to interpretations or suggestions, and follow through on agreed-on plans. He commented fairly frequently on the beneficial results he believed were due to therapy and generally seemed pleased with his therapeutic experience.

> The client entered therapy with the expectation of being provided with answers for all her problems. When this was not forthcoming, she became belligerent and expressed her dissatisfaction with therapy. She seemed more interested in having an opportunity to describe her problems in detail than in attempting to examine them or begin any programs

to change her situation or behavior. Any interruption of her complaints resulted in antagonistic comments about me and therapy. Generally, she was dissatisfied with the treatment she received and made little progress.

A major emphasis of the termination report must be a discussion of the events surrounding the end of treatment: the client's reasons for terminating; your impressions of the situation; your actions and responses as well as the client's; and any plans and suggestions for the future. All this information will be invaluable to a future therapist who may have to continue from where you left off. For example:

The client terminated therapy because he wanted to enter marriage counseling with his wife, and we decided that this would be best handled by a new, "neutral" therapist. The timing of termination seemed appropriate to me, because he had reached new understanding of his problems and was ready to begin an active program to improve his marriage.

The client terminated therapy because she said that she could not afford the sessions. There had been no change in her financial situation, and she refused to discuss a different payment schedule. At the time of termination therapeutic discussions had begun to focus on the client's feelings toward men, which seemed to be a very anxiety-provoking area for her. I expressed my opinion that there were important issues to be dealt with and that possibly she was leaving therapy in order to avoid dealing with her mistrust of men and general fear of intimacy. However, the client was adamant in terminating. She was encouraged to reapply for treatment if she changed her mind.

A brief abstract or synopsis of treatment is often included with the termination summary. This is convenient to have available, because a brief summary of therapy is often supplied in response to a client's authorization for the release of information. For example:

The client, a thirty-seven-year-old married white male, was seen for twelve therapy sessions between July 6 and

October 12, 1976. He sought therapy because of feelings of depression primarily centering around his marriage. The focus of therapy was on increasing his awareness of the factors contributing to his unhappiness. The client developed considerable understanding of the contributing problems, and on the basis of this new perspective decided to seek marriage counseling with his wife. As he became more aware of his problems and feelings and began to make some decisions about his marriage his mood improved considerably.

In summary, although record keeping often seems like unimportant busy work arbitrarily imposed by compulsive administrative staff, it is not fruitless effort but an important part of both the client's treatment and your training. Report writing forces you continually to examine and focus on the course of treatment and the client's progress. Good records also provide invaluable information to others who will have contact with your client. The time invested in keeping good records will pay important dividends to both you and your client.

Part IV

Adapting to other treatment contexts

13
Cotherapy

Why do cotherapy?

Working conjointly with another therapist has considerable appeal for the beginning therapist facing the complex
and difficult task of seeing two or more clients together,
which can be overwhelming when you have limited skills
and many fears about your capabilities. You may not feel
sufficiently competent to handle a couple or a group alone,
but may well feel more confident combining your efforts
with those of another therapist. The cotherapy situation
allows you the opportunity to share the burden of responsibility. If nothing else, there is solace in facing a difficult
and sometimes fearful task with another person. A beginner often will feel less pressure because the demands are
reduced for either of the cotherapists to be actively interacting or fully attentive at any given time. Pressure is also
reduced when problem solving and decision making are
shared.

Clearly, cotherapy is not without its problems and
drawbacks. These are best understood by looking at the
frequent reluctance of experienced therapists to do cotherapy. For one, the experienced therapist has often developed a working style with which he or she is comfortable; the intrusion of another therapist requires some
adaptation of this style. Working with another person
also demands that you give up some of your freedom to
operate in the manner you feel is most effective or com-

fortable for you. The pace of therapy and the timing of interventions will be affected. For example, you as a therapist may find it most useful to bypass a question your client has raised. It may be disconcerting to find your cotherapist pursuing the question.

To do cotherapy well you must be able to work intimately with another person. Experienced therapists most often work alone with their clients in the privacy of their offices. Only infrequently do they come under the observation of another professional. Cotherapy requires blending the working skills of two professionals in a complementary way. You must feel comfortable with your cotherapist and must reveal feelings and reactions that you have traditionally kept private. You also need to trust the professional skill and judgment of another person. As you can see, the development of an effective, shared working style can be personally taxing and very time-consuming. It is no wonder that many experienced therapists opt to work alone.

Many of these issues may be less of a problem for you, the beginner, in that your therapy style is in its formative stages and may be more open to modification and compromise. However, beginners initially underestimate the complexity of cotherapy and later experience some severe problems. For example:

> A talkative student and a quiet one who were working together as cotherapists dismissed rather lightly the supervisor's concerns about equal participation in an upcoming intake interview. They claimed to be aware of this problem and felt they could prevent any difficulty. During the first interview the more active therapist totally dominated the interaction, with almost no input from the quieter student. Both trainees left the interview upset and angry about the other's behavior and their own inability to modify their natural styles.

Whether you are a beginner or an experienced therapist, there are a range of advantages to doing cotherapy in the multiple-client situation. Cotherapy has also been done with a single client (multiple therapists), but it can be overpowering for a client and provide a minimum therapeutic advantage unless done by therapists very experienced with the technique. In working with couples, families, and groups, cotherapy can provide a greater degree of flexibility than is available when the individual therapist works alone. This approach allows the introduction of therapists of each sex, a marked advantage in many situations. The availability of two therapists permits more variation in technique, style, and therapist roles. For example, in sex therapy each of the cotherapists can take an advocacy role with the same-sex client. This approach allows the therapist to align himself or herself with the special concerns and fears of one client while knowing that the cotherapist will be performing the same function for the other member of the couple. A single therapist would have an extremely difficult time trying to provide such an advocacy role without destroying the balance of the therapeutic situation.

This greater flexibility is also seen in the broader range of roles the therapist can assume. You will be presented with opportunities to model a wide range of behaviors that can make a therapeutic contribution. These include demonstrating communication patterns, settling disagreements, and making decisions. In addition, you will find it easier to utilize some specific treatment techniques, such as role playing, psychodrama, and fight training, when you have a partner with whom to demonstrate or share responsibilities.

The presence of a cotherapist allows each of you a much greater opportunity to monitor and observe what is going on in the therapy environment. It is difficult, and often impossible, to become involved in an intense interaction with one client and still monitor adequately what is happening to each of the other clients. Trusting that your cotherapist will provide this backup support allows you to become more intensively involved with some portion of what is happening. It also permits the luxury of taking some therapeutic risks that would be very difficult if you were working alone. You can challenge, criticize, or support in ways that would be injudicious without the presence of a cotherapist. The additional person can balance the communication and be aware of your excesses and compensate for them. For example, you may wish to confront strongly a couple's recent resistance to working on their problems. Working alone you might temper your response out of concern for alienating or totally discouraging your clients. However, in cotherapy you could respond strongly knowing that your cotherapist can add balance, if necessary, by pointing out the clients' earlier efforts and successes.

In addition to the value of one cotherapist counterbalancing the other, considerable therapeutic power can be generated by the therapists joining together with a combined focus of concern or support. When an individual therapist responds to a client, there is a greater opportunity to avoid or discount the opinion or comments of the therapist. When confronted by two therapists both in agreement, the client will most often have to give the therapists' feedback greater consideration.

The added flexibility and power of cotherapy can be particularly helpful in dealing with clients who are more difficult and resistive to treatment. You will often find that difficult clients will join forces against a single therapist. In such circumstances the sharing of responsibility can prevent the cotherapists from becoming overly discouraged and will generally make it easier to maintain control over the therapy sessions. Although such cases will still be troublesome, cotherapy will reduce some of the pressures and enable more powerful interventions that can increase the chances of success. For example:

> Two cotherapists were engaged in counseling a couple with severe marital problems. Nearly each time a therapist would make a confrontative comment both members of the couple would attack the therapist for being too vague and unclear. These reactions would serve to dis-

174

tract from the substance of the therapist's remarks. When handled solely by the therapist immediately involved in the interaction, an impasse would occur. However, progress would sometimes be made when the cotherapist would intervene as the "third party," point out the process of avoidance, and join forces with his cotherapist by agreeing with the initial comments. This strengthening of the cotherapist position made it difficult for the clients to continue to deflect the focus from their own behavior.

Choosing cotherapists

In your training you will probably have an opportunity to do some cotherapy. You may choose a cotherapist or have one assigned to you. If the latter is the case, you will probably have some say in assessing whether the team is workable. We will look at some of the factors to consider in choosing an appropriate cotherapist. We have found that it is generally best to have both a male and a female cotherapist, if possible. The client unit will probably have a mixed-sex composition, and having a therapist of each sex provides better balance, more effective models, and a fuller range of understanding of diverse problems.

Cotherapy with a more experienced therapist. Two cotherapy training models are frequently used: first, the pairing of a less experienced person with someone of considerably more skill; and second, the pairing of two beginning therapists of approximately equivalent training and skill. In the first model the mixing of beginner and experienced therapist allows the beginning therapist an opportunity to have a cotherapy experience in a relatively sheltered setting and to be able to observe and learn from a more skilled person. This type of pairing also introduces greater skill and experience directly into the session, rather than through supervision alone.

This approach is not without hazards, however. The discrepancy in skill often results in an uneven division of labor and responsibility. The less experienced person can defer to the point that the treatment becomes a solo practitioner performance, and the added therapeutic effectiveness of the cotherapy approach is lost. Clients become acutely aware of significant skill and authority differences and often respond accordingly. This approach can be used effectively, but requires considerable planning and discussion beforehand to counter potential problems. An example:

> A very authority-conscious couple were seen by an experienced therapist and a therapist in training. The couple insisted on calling one of the therapists "Doctor," while calling the other by first name, despite the equivalency of titles. The differential manner of addressing the two therapists was accompanied by a similar weighting of the comments of each of the therapists and constituted a major therapeutic problem.

Cotherapy with another student. Although it may seem attractive to have an experienced cotherapist to lean on and observe, we find that cotherapy with two beginning therapists is more practical, frequently presents fewer problems, and develops better basic skills. This approach is also not without its complexities. First, only rarely do beginners have equal experience or skill levels. It will be necessary to balance strengths and weakness so as to have a pair of therapists who complement each other and provide the array of therapeutic skills necessary for effective treatment. Doing therapy with another beginner who has essentially equal strengths and a similar style can lead to omissions and deficits in technique. Although the goal of cotherapy is for the therapists to complement each others' strengths, opposite qualities can also lead to difficulties. For example, pairing a student who is verbally aggressive with a shy, quiet person can create almost insurmountable problems. The quiet person must use the opportunity to strive toward an approximately equal verbal contribution. The verbally aggressive therapist needs to refrain from dominating and to allow

176

pauses during which the partner can initiate. The use of two novice cotherapists demands a commitment to honest, critical evaluation of each other's work and to the development of new skills necessary to attain an effective working relationship.

Cotherapy with friends. Beginning therapists often find it attractive to do cotherapy with individuals with whom they already have a comfortable interpersonal relationship. The natural choice is often a friend. Students typically assume that the comfort and sharing found in a friendship will generalize to therapy. Yet the cotherapy situation calls for a different kind of interaction and an existing relationship may interfere with developing a complementary working style. In addition, some premises of friendship can become barriers to mutual learning and professional growth. For example, it is not unusual in friendships to maintain an unstated pact to protect one another; this may interfere with open constructive criticism. Cotherapy is sufficiently complex by itself that it is best not burdened with the entanglements of a friendship. As a beginning therapist you may work better with someone with whom you have some acquaintance, but not a close friendship. You must know a potential cotherapist well enough to decide if there is some interpersonal ease, the ability to communicate, and the potential for trust. People who find each other clearly abrasive or untrustworthy will ultimately make a poor cotherapy team.

Preparing to work together

Getting acquainted with your cotherapist is of prime importance. Spending time together discussing your therapeutic experiences, orientation, style, and strengths and weaknesses is a necessity *before* you ever step into the therapy room. As essential as sharing information about yourselves is developing a reasonably equal information base about your clients. Equalization of treatment responsibility almost always requires equal knowledge about the clients and a shared understanding of therapeutic goals and the techniques to be used. All too often when one cotherapist depends on the other for his or her knowledge of the specific treatment approach to be used, that person increasingly relegates himself or herself to a secondary role in the treatment. This affects not only the relationship between the therapists, but also the relationship between clients and therapists. These preparations and briefings should precede your seeing the clients. Development of this new cotherapy relationship will likely require much planning time spent between the cotherapists by themselves as well as extensive preparation time together with the case supervisor.

It is inevitable that difference in opinion, treatment style, and assessment of the clients will come into focus during these discussions. Beginning therapists tend to minimize the importance of these differences. However, if they are not dealt with they can become very troublesome. Differences must be identified early and some consideration given to how they will be handled. Cotherapists need not always agree, but they must have a strategy for handling their disagreements. When discussing your disagreements, it is important to be able to differentiate substantive from stylistic differences. The latter are inevitable, and it is to be hoped that you will respect such differences even though they can be annoying. Substantive differences can be most important. For example, a major conflict can occur if therapists treating a couple strongly disagree as to whether the clients' past grievances should become a major focus of therapy. Major cotherapist differences, or any other significant problem that arises, require the assistance of a third party – the case supervisor. Although the use of two cotherapists provides a system of checks and balances that does not exist with an individual therapist, the complexity of the relationship makes the intervention of the supervisor extremely important.

The final step in preparation for the first cotherapy ses-

178

sion involves planning strategy and, in particular, deciding on a division of responsibilities. Although experienced cotherapists can often begin working with clients without much consideration for these details, a lack of preparation among beginners can lead to great silences, awkwardness, and uncomfortable glances. Having a well-planned, shared framework for the first session can help you start treatment smoothly.

Working outside the session

The complexity of cotherapy and the demands of maintaining an effective, complementary relationship require much work between treatment sessions. After working together for a long time, seasoned therapists are able to minimize time spent outside of sessions, but even they cannot operate without it. We recommend in addition to regular supervision that the cotherapists meet before and after each session to prepare for the meetings and then to debrief. Meeting before sessions allows the therapists to be sure they have a shared frame of reference about the upcoming meeting, have considered unresolved matters, and have reviewed goals and strategies. After the session you have the opportunity to share impressions about all levels of interaction: client–client, client–therapist, and therapist–therapist interaction. Good cotherapy cannot be conducted without your feeling free to give your cotherapist honest feedback about his or her performance and sharing feelings about the encounter. The complexity of the situation demands a *problem-hunting* orientation. Was there balance? Were there any problems between the therapists? Did there seem to be any disruptive alliances? Supervision allows a more in-depth look at the session, particularly to identify issues of which the therapists are not aware.

Working within the session

Working with a cotherapist facilitates certain therapeutic efforts and complicates others. The manner in which you interact with your colleague during the session is critical. You present your clients with an important interpersonal model to observe that becomes an active psychotherapeutic ingredient. In addition to the interaction of the cotherapists, the interaction between clients and therapists is also very important. Both cotherapist– and client–therapist interaction will be examined in this section.

Between cotherapists. Communicating with one's cotherapist in the session is an entirely new realm for beginning therapists. You will probably feel extremely awkward. You may be confused about how to address one another and how to refer to your cotherapist when talking with clients. There are many options, but it can be useful to address each other in your accustomed way, using first names, and when talking to the clients refer to the cotherapist by the name used in the introduction – for example, "Miss Jones." Beginning therapists are consistently reluctant to talk directly with their cotherapist during sessions. Sometimes therapists go through the first few meetings without saying anything to one another. However, an important ingredient in cotherapy is the demonstration of how people reach a consensus, disagree, share responsibility, and solve problems. This requires that cotherapists readily discuss matters, check out impressions, and share concerns with one another during the sessions. In fact, one effective method of communicating with clients in a manner that diminishes defensiveness is to discuss your concerns about them with your cotherapist during the session. An example:

> One member of a cotherapy team tried to help a client recognize that her frequent difficulties with fatigue and illness might be related to her current life stresses. Repeated attempts failed; the client would immediately deny this possibility and restate that she had simply been ill. The therapist turned to his cotherapy colleague and stated, "I really feel bogged down talking with Mary about the possible relationship of her continuing fatigue and illness and problems at home. She seems unwilling to consider how

these frequent symptoms may be related to her difficulties
in handling stressful circumstances."

The decision making you do in the therapy situation will
include a wide range of matters, from when the next appointment will be to whether therapy should be discontin-
ued. Some decisions are best made away from the sessions
after discussing the matter thoroughly with your cotherapist. Other decisions can and should be made during the
sessions; some very weighty matters cannot wait for
another session. In attempting to resolve an issue with
your cotherapist it is important that you clearly state your
thinking on the matter and offer your recommendation. It
is also important to check out your cotherapist's impressions, recommendations, and reactions to your solution.
Both therapists need not agree initially but should resolve
their differences and reach a mutual decision. Some disagreement can be useful; but it can become destructive
when frustration, competition, and hostility begin to surface in the relationship. When therapists sense they are
having serious problems in reaching agreement, it is im-
perative that they move their problems to another arena,
beyond the therapy room. There is no question that the
cotherapy situation does open the door for a variety of serious cotherapist relationship problems. People can become
competitive and vie for the support and admiration of
their clients. One therapist can undermine another's efforts. Close and frequent self-monitoring and feedback
from a supervisor are vital to avoid these counterproductive tendencies.

Between client and therapist. Cotherapy also provides a
situation in which you can carefully monitor the client–
therapist interaction. You can best observe how a client
interacts with therapist when you are not directly involved in that interaction. This more objective view will
enable you to notice actions or gestures that may be
missed by the other therapist and to identify confusions
that should be clarified.

Because of the sheer number of people involved, the relationships and alliances among all the participants in cotherapy become very complicated. The alliances that become established between individuals can have an important effect on the progress and outcome of therapy. It is essential that the therapists observe and identify these. In working with couples it frequently occurs that one of the clients will side with the therapists, attempting to develop an alliance with the therapists against the spouse and thereby gain an advantage. You may also find clients joining together and aligning themselves against the therapists. Therapists themselves are not immune from falling into unproductive alliances. A therapist may move to an adversary relationship with his or her cotherapist to protect a client from what he or she perceives as unfair comments. Any alliance that detours treatment from its goals is a problem. Cotherapists must be observant of all alliances that develop, determine to what degree they may interfere with therapy, and deal with them effectively.

Your experience with cotherapy will provide the opportunity to observe and encounter some of the more subtle and complex aspects of therapy. Although this approach in some ways reduces pressures on the beginner, it requires introduction to some of the more sophisticated therapy skills.

14
Children and families

Although some beginning clinicians are initially more comfortable handling child or family cases than treating adults, others are much more anxious about therapy with children. Students may be unsure of their therapeutic skills with adults, but at least they feel they can talk to them. An adult outpatient will usually act in socially acceptable ways, whereas a child's behavior may be less predictable. Adults come into your office when asked, sit in their chairs, and usually answer your questions appropriately. On the other hand, children sometimes cry when you greet them, refuse to come into your office, or are unable to sit quietly in a chair for more than a few minutes at a time. Although the therapist's worst fears are rarely realized, there are unique problems in child cases that you may find troublesome.

We consider treating children sufficiently different from therapy with typical adult clients that this entire chapter will be devoted to describing some needed changes in your interviewing techniques and some additions to your repertoire of therapeutic skills. However, it should be clearly understood that this chapter cannot by itself provide you with the necessary information for adequately assessing and treating a child. Numerous books have been written solely describing procedures for treating children and families. The aim of this chapter is to provide the beginner with a brief overview of some of the common problems and differences to be aware of in child therapy and to present a few pointers that may be useful in your initial child or family therapy interviews. The bulk of your training for therapy with children will come from your teachers, supervisors, and specialized reading on this topic.

Differences in expectations about therapy

In earlier chapters we have described some of the general goals of assessment and therapy interviewing that apply to both child and adult cases. Briefly, in child cases you will need to acquire detailed information about the presenting problems and relevant history regarding onset and development of these problems. You will also usually want some historical information about the child and other family members as well as a description of the family's current life situation. Your assessment of the case will be derived from the questions you ask and your observations of the child and other family members, as we've discussed earlier.

However, you may have to alter your strategy to accommodate the differences involved in interviewing children and families. Unfortunately, there are no hard-and-fast rules dictating the exact changes that will be needed in all the situations you are likely to encounter. For instance, the way you interview a child depends on his or her age, behavior, and level of maturity. Obviously, there are great differences in how you will relate to a six-year-old and to a sixteen-year-old, although there may be minimal differences between a sixteen-year-old and a twenty-one-year-old "adult." The expectations that children and parents have for therapy are frequently different from those typical with individual adult cases. We describe some of these common differences and discuss some possible ways to respond.

Preparing the child for therapy. Many of your initial efforts in a child or family case are aimed at dealing with the special problems that arise because the person with the identified problems, the child, has usually not independently chosen to seek help. Most likely therapy has been arranged by the parent or guardian to deal with problems that others in the environment have identified. In contrast, most adult clients view themselves as having some difficulties about which they expect to be asked. This difference has many implications for how to proceed.

To begin with, you should be prepared to deal with the fact that the child may not understand who you are, why he or she has come to see you, and what you will do. Understandably, this can make a child anxious and distrustful. Preparing the child for the events of therapy can prevent these fears from becoming exaggerated. In fact, parents often ask what they should tell the child about therapy. We believe it is valuable to schedule a first session with the parents (or guardian) alone to discuss this issue. It can be reassuring to an uncertain parent as well as useful in paving the way for a nonthreatening first contact with the child. However, one must weigh the positive aspects of meeting without the child against the possibility that he or she may learn of it and feel that the adults are plotting together. If this is a serious concern, much of the information can be conveyed adequately over the phone.

Although there are always exceptions, we believe that parents can be fairly direct in explaining to a child their reasons for seeking therapy. It is likely that the child is already aware that the parents are concerned about something. It will come as no surprise if the parents again openly express their concerns and explain that they are going to talk to someone who specializes in helping people with these types of problems. The parents should attempt to make clear to the child that the therapist will ask the family members about themselves and the problems they are experiencing. If any other procedures are planned, such as testing, the child should also be told about them in a way he or she can understand. It is important that the child not be misled into expecting that the meeting will be just like school or play. When younger children are told about therapy, it is also a good idea for the parents not to use the word *doctor,* because this may evoke fears of getting a shot or having a tooth pulled.

A first meeting with the parent(s) alone will certainly provide valuable information about the case and can be useful in your preparation for interviewing the child and other family members. On the basis of the initial information you may even discover (1) that therapy is not indicated, (2) that the child's problems are secondary to severe marital difficulties, or (3) that therapy should proceed *without* the child's involvement. For example,

> A husband, fifty-one years old, and a wife, forty-three, wanted to make an appointment for their seven-year-old son because they thought he was hyperactive. They were bothered by his "constantly moving around," but stated that otherwise they had no problems with their son. To the therapist, the son's activity level, as described by the parents, seemed normal for a boy that age. Both a school and home visit confirmed this initial impression. It was therefore decided that therapy sessions should include only the parents and focus on developing more appropriate expectations regarding normal behavior for a seven-year-old.

Even after you have discussed with the parents what the child should be told about therapy, you can never be sure what was actually communicated. Consequently, it is useful early in the assessment period to meet with the entire family and ask each person what he or she expects from therapy. This provides you with an opportunity to correct any misconceptions and make any needed preparatory remarks. Be sure to gear your explanations to the child's level of understanding.

You should not only ask the child why he or she thinks therapy has been initiated, but also gather the opinions of all the family members present. This will allow you both to acquire everyone's perspective on the problems and to observe the communication patterns within the family.

186

Besides inquiring about the specific presenting problem, it is also a good procedure to ask everyone if there are any other difficulties in their lives, individually or as a family.

Dealing with an uncooperative or distrusting child. Many children or adolescents seen for therapy are referred by a court or social agency. Although the issue of trust is important in all cases, it is critical when the client has been ordered to see you. You may be faced with a client who is angry, distrustful, and resentful. These feelings may be understandable, but it does not make your interview any easier if your client is hostile, is unmotivated to change, and denies any problems.

As a general rule, if you believe the issue of trust is likely to be a primary concern for any client, this should be discussed. If your client does not bring up the issue, you should. In discussing this with a client it is important not to make any demands for immediate trust, such as offhandedly saying, "You can trust me." It is better to recognize and admit that the client has no reason at this point to trust you, but that in time you hope to establish a relationship within which the sharing of personal thoughts and feelings will be possible.

If a resistant or uncooperative child is being seen because of illegal activities, you may not wish to press for the details of the crime. He or she may fear that you will repeat everything to the parents or the referring agency. In time the client may feel more comfortable talking about those problems, but there will certainly be other things to talk about. You should deal with legal problems in a straightforward way, acknowledging that you know about them and in a matter-of-fact way asking the client to describe the situation. It is wise to be cautious and not push clients already coerced into therapy to talk about themselves or specific problem areas if they are unwilling to do so.

You also should not feel that the client's problems have to be solved right from the start. It will take longer than usual to build trust and rapport, and these are sufficient initial goals. On the other hand, you should not let yourself be "conned" by a client in the interests of establishing trust. If you think a client is deceiving you, you can acknowledge this without conveying reproach. Lastly, it is critically important to avoid making any promises to a client that you cannot keep, such as saying that everything you are told is confidential when this is not the case. Both you and the client must be realistic about the constraints of the situation. To convey anything else would be to do the client a great injustice and undermine any hope of developing a trusting relationship.

Preparing the parents for therapy. Thus far we have primarily concentrated on potential problems arising from a child's expectations or ignorance about what will occur in therapy. However, you will also frequently encounter difficulties because parents are unprepared for their involvement. Adults often assume that the entire focus of assessment and therapy will be on the child. They may resent being asked about personal matters. The attitude, whether spoken or unspoken, is, "I brought my son in because he has problems. Why do you want to talk to me?" This does not imply that everyone will be uncooperative or resentful; however, it is useful initially to lay the groundwork for your interview by explaining the type of information you will need and why it is necessary. You might preface your questions with the following statement: "In order to understand what is happening with your child, I need to know certain kinds of information about each of you and how your family interacts."

This approach does not always ensure success. Some parents will adamantly refuse to disclose any information about themselves or their marital relationship. If this occurs you will have to decide how important the parents' information is to your assessment and treatment. If you think it is vital, you may have to tell the parents that it is futile for you to proceed further without their coopera-

tion. If you believe you can do an adequate job of helping
the child without personal information from the parents,
it is probably best to continue without pushing the issue
and further alienating them.

Of course, many parents have an appropriate and positive attitude toward therapy. However, you should be prepared for a wide variety of attitudes, some of which may
be very unproductive. For example, some parents will be
angry at their child about his or her problem behaviors
and expect you to be punitive. Others may react with
feelings of failure and guilt and will either see you as a
potential critic or want you to affirm that they have done
all that could be done. They may also be defensive or
resistant because of being threatened by your success
with the child – which would confirm their own failure.

In addition, when dealing with families you are much
more likely to be asked for advice. Students often feel
threatened by parents who demand an immediate opinion about problems – for example, whether a child should
be given an allowance or be expected to earn it, whether
the child is old enough to date, and so forth. This presents a delicate situation for the therapist. You will not
want to impose your own child-rearing values on your
clients, nor do you want to become identified with one
family member's point of view. It is important to refrain
from offering your opinions until you understand the situation thoroughly and have carefully thought through
the consequences of your advice. It is generally wise to
be extremely cautious in such situations.

Parents differ widely in their views about child rearing
and acceptable behavior. What one family will tolerate is
very disturbing to another. Should you therefore agree to
therapy goals even if you believe the parents' expectations are unrealistic? These are difficult judgments to
make. You have to wrestle with each case individually.
Appropriate goals may be arrived at through gradual negotiation with the parents about their expectations and
the consequences of these standards for the child. You

may find that child and family cases initially tap your diplomatic talents as much as your therapeutic ones.

Communicating with children

Thus far we have focused on the effects of differences in the expectations of family members in regard to therapy. When interviewing children you should also be aware of the child's level of intellectual and emotional funtioning and conduct your interviews within these restraints. It is particularly important when dealing with younger children to remember that you cannot talk to them in the same way you do to an adult. Students often recognize this but, as a result, seem either condescending or overly friendly. You have to assess what a child can understand and communicate at that level. Your vocabulary should be simple, and questions should be phrased concretely. Children do not have an adult's abilities to respond to abstract concepts or to remember long, complicated questions. Most often it is best to ask brief questions that call for descriptions of situations or events, rather than to ask complicated questions about feelings or opinions, particularly in the initial stages of therapy. A child may say nothing in answer to a question or may give an incomprehensible answer; frequently you simply have to accept less verbal clarity with children and not waste time attempting repeatedly to pin down some specific point.

Students who are accustomed to asking questions and collecting verbal information may find themselves at a loss. Particularly with young or anxious children, beginning the session by talking can be quite unproductive. You will get very little information and will probably make yourself and the client even more anxious. Using some nonverbal medium, such as drawing, structured games, or unstructured play, can be very helpful in developing rapport, reducing anxiety, and facilitating verbal self-disclosure.

It is particularly difficult to elicit information about a

child's feelings by asking questions. The child may not even have the vocabulary to express these concepts. You will need to be flexible, creative, and persistent in your attempts. You might propose how you would feel in a situation and ask if that sounds similar to the way the child feels. This may lead him or her to talk in greater detail about personal feelings. Or you might describe a situation similar to the child's and ask how other children would feel or act in that situation. Some child therapists use play as a setting for children to talk about the feelings of dolls or imaginary characters in various situations, including some analogous to the child's life.

It is important to remember that most children are unaccustomed to labeling negative feelings, especially anger or fear, in relation to adults. They are simply not used to telling one adult that they are angry at another adult (e.g., parents or teachers). They may have been taught that this is wrong, that they *shouldn't* feel angry at "Daddy" or "Mommy," or that they are too big to be afraid.

Not only do you have to be careful about the complexity of the words and thoughts you use with children, but your manner of phrasing is also very important. Children often respond to the literal meaning of your statements and not to their figurative meaning. If you are not careful about how you say things, a child may take you literally at your word. For instance, one of the most common errors that beginners make with children is to phrase statements or commands as questions. If you say to a typical adult client, "Would you like to come into my office now?" they will almost always follow you into your office. If you say this to a child, he is very likely to answer, "No." If you offer a child an option, you must be prepared to allow him or her to take it. Otherwise the child will be unlikely to trust what you say from that point on.

Similarly, you have to be careful about the use of humor, which often involves the figurative use of words. Teasing or making jokes with children is a fine art. If a therapist knows what he or she is doing, it can lighten the atmosphere and facilitate the interview. However, if it is not done well, it can result in a child feeling hurt, upset, confused, and antagonistic toward you. We advise a cautious approach unless you are experienced in working with children. In fact, the judicious use of words in your statements to and about the child is always important. Children are often very sensitive and interpret many statements as being critical of them, especially when pertaining to their problems, and their feelings may inadvertently be hurt by careless words or comments.

Because children have not developed socially appropriate ways of dealing with emotions, they are more apt to show overt signs of stress and act out their feelings. An adult may feel like hiding in a corner because he or she is afraid or embarrassed; a child may actually try to hide. The same type of overt expression can occur for any other emotion a child feels. If a child is afraid, he or she may cry; if angry, he or she may throw a tantrum. These kinds of reactions may not be frequent, but you should be prepared for them. Beginners who are insecure about their professional competence may have difficulty tolerating children acting in childish ways. It will be important for you to learn to accept the child's feelings and provide support if needed, yet at the same time set clear and firm expectations about acceptable behavior for therapy sessions.

You must also remember that a child does not have the attention span or the tolerance for frustration that an adult has. Children cannot talk about their problems for as long as an adult. When you interview children, their anxiety and frustration during the session should be carefully monitored. If a child begins to fidget or seems unduly distracted after talking to you for a while, it may be time to change the focus of the interview or to intersperse some other, less demanding activities, such as drawing or play. These other activities may also be important parts of your assessment and therapeutic procedures, but they can be alternated with more stressful discussions of the child's problems or life situation. At times you may have to schedule a number of brief meetings with a child rather than a single longer interview.

Assessment of children's problems

Besides the usual evaluation that occurs as a function of your interviewing with children and family members, child cases often include additional types of assessment procedures. Frequently, parents seek therapy because of questions regarding a child's school performance and intellectual capacity, and intelligence tests will provide critical information for your evaluation. At other times tests that measure other aspects of psychological functioning may prove a useful adjunct in your diagnosis of a problem.

Testing will also give you the opportunity to see the child alone; however, you may encounter some problems when it is time to separate the child from the parents. The child may cry, cling to the parent, or refuse to come to the testing room. We believe it is valuable initially to see the child together with the person(s) who brought him or her. This may make the child more comfortable and lessen the fear of being alone with you. It is helpful to prepare the child for testing by explaining what will happen and how long you expect to be. If you are going to another room, a parent may have to accompany you as you walk over. In extreme cases a parent may need to stay in the room while you test, play with, or talk to the child. The way a child responds to being separated from the parents is, of course, valuable information to be noted in your assessment, as is the difference in the child's behavior in the presence versus the absence of the parents.

In child cases you have the opportunity of observing a great deal of a client's significant environment by making a home or school visit. Although environmental factors are important with all clients, the possibility of controlling so many aspects of the environment is unique to child cases.

Home visits. Parents' reports of a child's behavior at home often are stereotyped, simple descriptions that do not provide you with the depth of information you need for an adequate assessment. Parents are not necessarily perceptive or accurate observers. Their view may also be distorted because of their notions of what is acceptable behavior for their child. By visiting the home you can acquire firsthand information about the child's interactions with parents and other family members. You will be able to observe the behaviors that have been labeled as problematic as well as the situations in which they occur. You may become aware of the function the child's deviant behavior serves in the family unit as you observe the consequences accruing to the problem behaviors. The opportunity will also be available to observe aspects of the child's behavior or family functioning that have not been mentioned but that may provide you with a different perspective. For instance, you may discover that the child engages in many appropriate behaviors that go unrecognized by the parents, and that only the few inappropriate behaviors are noticed.

When visiting the home you can observe how all the family members relate to each other and the characteristic qualities of these interactions. There are often other difficulties in a family where a child has been identified as the problem. By observing the family functioning as a unit you may be alerted to other difficulties that may later emerge or hinder the progress of therapy. You may also become aware of the potential effects of your interventions on the child and the family unit and prepare for (and possibly prevent) troublesome ramifications resulting from these changes.

School visits. Problems in school are frequently either the primary complaint that brings children to therapy or else an associated problem. School personnel have important information and opinions about the child that you will need to assess the case. Most useful will be information about the child's behavior and academic performance in school and his or her relationships with peers and authority figures other than the parents. This is critical information that may sometimes be surprising and may contradict what the parents have told you.

When arranging a school visit you should always confer first with the principal and the teacher about a time that will allow you to observe the most relevant sample of the child's behavior. The child should be told beforehand that you may come to visit the school room some day. Do not surprise him or her by appearing unexpectedly. However, it is best to leave the time and day of your visit unspecified to avoid having the child prepare for you in some atypical way (like being sick that day).

It is very important to spend considerable time before a school (or home) visit deciding what approach you will take and what information you will need. The time to decide what you will ask the teacher is not when you are walking up to the school or talking on the phone. If school problems are a major area of difficulty, you will be working closely with the teacher in developing and coordinating a treatment plan. You must conduct your contacts with school personnel in a careful and respectful manner. Teachers are professionals who have valuable opinions and observations. They may also be directly responsible for implementing therapeutic interventions. Good communication is important from the beginning so that teachers have input into the assessment process and treatment planning and later fully understand the proposed treatment procedures. If a treatment plan is different from what a teacher knows about or has experience with, time and effort have to be taken to explain the procedures fully and to reach an agreement both the teacher and therapist accept. A treatment program in the school can only be successfully implemented if the teacher understands it, agrees with it, and then carries it out.

Treatment of children's problems

As with adult therapy, different theoretical orientations to child cases will lead to different treatment methods. For instance, some child therapists always treat the entire family, some see only the child, and others meet mostly with the parents and rarely see the child. However, regardless of theoretical orientation, some potential difficulties commonly emerge in child cases, and it is prudent to be alert to them.

Some parents want you to cure the child without their changing or investing any of their time or effort in therapy. This bias may be so strong that the parents will refuse to cooperate with you in a treatment plan that includes their involvement. In this case you are faced with the decision of seeing the child alone or explaining to the parents that you do not believe you can be of service to them, and why. In making this decision you will have to weigh costs and benefits to the child, and supervisory assistance will be needed to make a good decision. As a general rule, the usefulness of seeing the child alone increases with the child's age. The older a child is, the more beneficial it may be to see a therapist independently. You may be able to provide support and guidance to a fifteen-year-old in leading his or her life that is not possible with a five-year-old, whose control over the environment is minimal.

When you are seeing family groups, your actions serve as a model of how to interact with the people involved. If you respect the opinion of everyone, including the children, this will be noticed and possibly modeled by those present. There is a tendency on the part of students to ignore children during a session, especially if a child is quiet or hard to talk to. The child may just sit while the therapist and the parents discuss the "child's problems."

This insensitivity can lessen the child's involvement and hamper the effectiveness of therapy, and it is a poor model for the parents.

Just as in all other types of therapy, you will develop a relationship with the people involved in a child or family case. You will like some and dislike others, trust some and distrust others. However, you must be careful to monitor your feelings so that they do not interfere with your ability to respond in a professional and therapeutic manner. For instance, it is easy to start disliking a child because you think he or she makes you look bad as a therapist. It is also easy to become emotionally overinvolved with the children you are seeing in therapy. At times they seem like helpless victims who are at the mercy of overbearing or insensitive parents. Beginning therapists often think they can "parent" the child better than parents and ally themselves with the child. When this happens you lose your effectiveness as a potential helping agent by alienating the parents. This also may not be fair to the child, who can become dependent on you, but whose continuation in therapy is up to the parents and whose real-life adjustment must ultimately be made in his or her own family.

Structuring the interview with children. It is important for the therapist to be in control of the general structure and flow of the session. Being in control involves maintaining behavior appropriate to the therapeutic setting as well as guiding the conversation into productive areas. You can expect children to test the limits of allowable behavior at some time during your sessions. If you respond in an equivocal or inconsistent fashion to their testing of the rules, it will reinforce their efforts to keep pressing the limits. Therefore it is best to be firm from the start.

In order to maintain control over a session you will have to act with an air of authority, be direct and firm in your statements, and be confident about what you are saying. If you are unsure about what to do, it is better to state this openly rather than trying to hide it from the client. The client will likely perceive your uncertainty and your attempt to conceal it. In fact, children may perceive and comment on your uncertainty more readily than adults, who tend to do what is socially appropriate and ignore it.

How you handle a child's testing of limits is only one example of the need to be careful about your responses to a child's behavior. It is easy inadvertently to establish troublesome behavior patterns. Your attention and responsivity to a child can be a powerful reward for both appropriate and inappropriate behavior. For example:

> A six-year-old boy was brought for therapy by his parents because the boy would not do what he was told and fought with other children at school. As soon as the boy entered the therapy room he began climbing on top of the table and pulling books down from a bookshelf. The therapist took hold of the boy and sat him in a chair. As soon as he let go, the boy repeated the pattern. This continued until the therapist was holding the boy in the chair for the remainder of the session.

> At the next session, after consulting with the supervisor, the therapist changed rooms to one that only had two chairs in it. He said that he had a few questions to ask and that when they were finished the boy could play with some toys. However, he would only talk to the boy while he was sitting down. The boy immediately got up and began walking around the room. This time the therapist did nothing but sit in his chair. After about twenty minutes the boy sat down in the chair and the therapist began talking to him. The boy got up again after a few minutes, and the therapist merely stopped talking. This happened a few more times, but finally the boy stayed in the chair for the rest of the session.

Beginning therapists are often troubled if a child acts inappropriately during a session, is noncompliant, or becomes very emotional. They think that this reflects their lack of ability and that if they were really good therapists the child would be a model of appropriate behavior. It would be much more realistic to expect a child with problems to display them in the session. The therapy setting is, in fact, a valuable opportunity for you to make a firsthand assessment of the problem and to derive hypotheses about what factors may be contributing to them.

Confidentiality. The rules of confidentiality that apply for adults do not apply to children. You cannot assure a child of complete confidentiality, because the parents have a legal right to be informed about any substantive issues that may affect the child's welfare. In court-referred cases the court may have similar rights to be informed about relevant issues discussed in therapy. Although this may make it initially somewhat more difficult to establish a trusting relationship, the issue can usually be discussed and negotiated. Parents often feel they have the right to know what occurs during therapy, because they are paying for it, whereas the child feels everything should be kept totally confidential. It may be possible to negotiate some mutually satisfactory agreement. For instance, the parents may agree to refrain from asking about what happens during therapy, or they may accept brief summary reports. You can at least assure a child that he or she will be told beforehand about anything you tell the parents. It is very important to discuss the issue of confidentiality early and to clarify with all parties what the ground rules will be. This can circumvent future problems and prevent potential feelings of betrayal.

Terminating therapy. There are some special considerations to keep in mind in terminating therapy with children. The manner in which you assess progress is different from that with adult clients. Children are often not able to tell you that they have changed or that the problems are resolved. This is especially true if they did not believe they had problems to begin with. You have to

199

measure progress by your own observations of the child and by the reports of family members, school personnel, or others.

Unfortunately, because children often have little control over the continuation of therapy, termination may occur without their being informed or consulted. In your planning of termination with a child it is important to remember that children do not have an adult's cognitive abilities to handle the ending of the relationship. Abruptly ending therapy may have a stronger emotional impact on a child than on an adult. However, a child is likely to be unable to describe his or her feelings about termination verbally and is more likely to respond primarily in an overt, emotional way. You will probably have to initiate most of the discussion on the child's feelings about the ending of therapy. It is important to emphasize, if it is the case, that the ending of therapy is due to the child's improvement or the resolution of problems and not to your dislike of him or her. If possible, it is advisable to stretch out the ending phase of therapy with children by scheduling sessions at increasingly longer intervals rather than by abruptly terminating after regular weekly sessions.

15

An epilogue: developing your skills

The process of learning to become a psychotherapist is a perplexing and difficult experience for many students. It requires a problem-solving approach and a set of skills that may be entirely new. Most students begin without much relevant experience, and previous training frequently does little to prepare them for this new role. In this book we have provided broad guidelines for therapy rather than specific prescriptions and stressed the importance of supervision. The traditional supervision of a beginner by an experienced professional is necessary to teach psychotherapeutic skills and to ensure an adequate level of service to the client.

Clinical skill attainment requires a level of involvement and change on the part of the student not generally expected elsewhere. It usually demands that you take risks by behaving in untried ways. It may require that you examine your own personality style, interpersonal relationships, and conflict areas. In addition to all this, you may also have to reveal personal problems or what you consider to be weaknesses to your supervisors and fellow trainees. This sort of exposure is often a novel experience for students and one that may make you feel quite vulnerable. Not surprisingly, few students initially feel comfortable in this situation.

Psychotherapy training requires a radical shift in learning style from what has generally proved to be successful for most students throughout their academic careers. Up until this point, students have been rewarded for solitary diligence and conscientiousness – reading, writing term papers, and taking examinations. Such an approach to learning is, of course, necessary to acquire a basic knowledge of personality theory and therapeutic schools of thought. However, it is not sufficient for learning how to interact with a client in a therapy session.

Suddenly students find themselves floundering in a critically important area where nothing they do seems to measure up and where the task itself is often incomprehensible. They interpret every client contact as a testing situation and go into it with the expectation that they must pass with flying colors. They need to be reminded constantly that it is both unwise and unrealistic to expect a high level of mastery at the outset when the only way to learn is by actually trying out the skill to be learned. Yet students in the mental health professions usually have a tremendous personal investment in demonstrating their proficiency in being able to interact with and assist others. As a consequence, failure in this area, whether real or imagined, can be particularly devastating.

In summary, the following four factors combine to make your clinical practicum training a particularly difficult experience: First, it requires learning entirely new skills that are critical to success in your career; second, it requires a change in your approach to learning; third, it involves personal vulnerability surrounding the exposure of your own personality and problems; and, fourth, the anticipation of failure in a key skill may make you more anxious and consequently less willing to take necessary risks to try out new ways of behaving.

In this chapter we will discuss a variety of methods you may use to improve and enlarge your clinical skills. Supervision is the prime tool available for your learning, but there are additional tools that will help you maximize your progress. We will first address ourselves to the supervisory process and later discuss other methods of skill attainment.

The supervision process

The student's dilemma. Learning to do psychotherapy under the supervision of an experienced clinician can be a personally rewarding and enriching experience for both you and your supervisor. You have the opportunity to expose your hopes and aspirations and share your growth and progress with another person. Unfortunately, however, the supervision situation also presents a conflict for the therapist in training. You are asked to reveal your anxieties, vulnerabilities, and weaknesses to a superior who generally has the responsibility of evaluating you. Your past academic experience has encouraged you to present instructors what you *know* and to remedy what you don't know on your own. Your ignorance is not the data of learning, as it is now in psychotherapeutic training. This conflict of interest often puts students in a bind, one they resolve only after gaining considerable trust in the supervisor.

Coupled with their concerns about looking bad, students often take criticism about their clinical abilities quite personally. This is not surprising, because much of therapy training involves examining the personality and interpersonal qualities of the student. It is much more difficult to accept a comment directed at your style of relating to other people than criticism about your style of writing in a term paper. The comments you will be receiving from clinical supervisors may have a direct impact on your personal confidence and self-esteem. From the supervisor's point of view as well, it is usually quite difficult to deliver these kinds of comments. The situation is made much worse when the trainee is either obviously devastated or defends himself or herself by explaining every move in great detail.

In addition to the difficulties built in by the special nature of your learning task, students tend to become further demoralized by comparing their own performance to the performance or apparent wisdom of their supervisors. This is truly a meaningless comparison. What you are doing is comparing yourself to someone who, when working with you, has the great advantage of hindsight and third-party objectivity. Your supervisor has a tremendous position of advantage, which few students recognize.

It will maximize your progress and make the experience much easier if you are able to put aside your concerns about evaluation and competititon with fellow students during clinical training. Very few students escape the experience of feeling awkward and not knowing what to do. This, added to their worries about offering adequate service to the client when they are as yet untrained, can make your beginning experiences quite trying. It sometimes helps to remember that you are learning a totally new skill and that it is unrealistic to expect yourself to perform well from the beginning. As in learning anything new, you will begin with a novice's level of competence.

The relationship you develop with your supervisor can be of great help to you in dealing with the problems you encounter in your training, both in regard to the client and to your own personal feelings about doing psychotherapy. Optimally you and your supervisor will develop a trusting and accepting relationship in which you will feel free to expose your vulnerabilities. The supervisor's task is both to assist you in your learning and to ensure that the client receives adequate service. By and large, supervisors are more concerned with your openness to learning and willingness to try out suggestions than with your beginning mistakes. At its best the supervisory relationship is an alliance in which you and your instructor mutually explore the client's problems and treatment, your therapy skills, and your personal reactions to training. This is an ideal notion and may be far from the reality of your situation. You will have numerous opportunities for seeking out supervisory and consultative relationships as your professional experience increases; you will find such interactions beneficial.

Handling differences of opinion. Many students are quite concerned about how to handle conflicts of opinion with the supervisor. They may disagree with the supervisor's theoretical orientation, value system, or choice of treatment approach. Contrary to what students expect, supervisors often welcome disagreement and the opportunity for an active dialogue with their trainees about clients. Many are not as wedded to their own ideas as students think, and they may appreciate and incorporate the students' comments and suggestions. A satisfactory consensus can usually be reached without hard feelings if disagreements are aired.

If you cannot reach an agreement with which both you and your supervisor are satisfied, a third party may be brought in who can be helpful in reconciling differences. However, even this may not result in satisfaction. When you and your supervisor have an unreconcilable disagreement about the treatment of your client, you will have to keep in mind that your supervisor bears the legal responsibility for the client, and, as such, must have the last word. The supervisor has the responsibility for maximizing the treatment situation for the client as well as for maximizing your training. Although it might be best for your learning to allow you to work things out on a trial-and-error basis, he or she has the ethical obligation of seeing that the client's treatment is adequate. This may mean that your supervisor will insist on a treatment approach that he or she believes will be in the client's best interests, even though you may disagree.

It may be helpful at such times to remind yourself that your training is not a time to be solidifying your own manner of approach. Instead you might view it as a time to explore new behaviors and new ways of looking at clinical problems. The ability to lend yourself to your supervisor's approach will reduce the strain on the supervisory relationship and may very well result in valuable new learning on your part.

How to maximize your learning through supervision. Although it may be painful to expose yourself to criticism from a supervisor, the supervision model is by far the most effective way of increasing your skills, particularly if your supervisor can actually observe you directly or through video tape. However, many students try to avoid direct scrutiny by their supervisor out of a fear of having their errors discovered.

Although we are sympathetic with how difficult it is to expose yourself to criticism, it is to your advantage to seek out direct feedback about your strengths and weaknesses in your actual interaction with the client. If you provide your supervisor with only the minimum amount of information about what happened in a therapy session, he or she will be able to be only minimally helpful. In addition, this attitude on your part will undoubtedly create tension in the supervisory relationship, with you trying to withhold information and the supervisor trying to ascertain what actually happened. Surprisingly enough, you may find out from your supervisor that you weren't as bad as you thought.

The value of supervision extends far beyond discussing the dynamics of the client's problems and how to implement a treatment plan. Although these are crucial elements, much of the actual clinical learning comes in closely examining what you communicate, verbally and nonverbally, the timing and clarity of your remarks, and the subtleties of your interpersonal interaction with the client. Many of these aspects of clinical interaction only become evident to you and your supervisor if you actually watch yourself in action.

Many students have an exaggerated fear of watching themselves on video tape or listening to an audio tape. They are terribly oversensitized to their mistakes and become preoccupied with anticipating them and with the humiliation of hearing the error all over again in the presence of an audience. Students sometimes allow their mistakes to assume too great an importance and overlook the more general impact of the session.

It's a shock to see or hear yourself on tape; you never look or sound quite like you expected. It is helpful to review your tapes alone prior to supervision. The shock is not quite so great, and you are less likely to be caught off guard by an unexpected criticism. By reviewing your own tapes alone before supervision you will give yourself the same advantage that the supervisor has – that of hindsight and improved objectivity. Although you are actually present during the therapy session, you rarely have the time to speculate much on your own behavior.

In and of itself, learning to monitor your progress is an important element of clinical training. Students generally learn in three stages. First, they learn to recognize their skills and errors after having them pointed out by someone else. Generally this is followed by an increased ability to analyze their own performance after the fact. Finally, they reach the point where they can evaluate their performance on the spot and correct or avoid errors within the session.

To get the most out of supervision it is also critical to bring your own feelings about and reactions to the client into the discussion. This area of information is generally available to you but unavailable to the supervisor unless you bring it up; yet it is the most important ingredient in improving your skills beyond the early stages. Your anxieties, sexual interest in the client, like or dislike, and the variety of other personal reactions you will have toward clients are critical information affecting treatment. All therapists, whether novice or expert, experience a wide range of feelings about their clients. This is the material of therapy, not a personal flaw, which many beginning students believe. For example, sexual feelings on your part may focus you on seductive behavior on the part of the client, which may be important to understanding his or her problems. It takes skill and confidence of a high order to be able to sort out your idiosyncratic responses from the more appropriate and relevant reactions to the client. You may never reach this level of skill unless you can talk about these issues in supervision.

A final critical issue in using supervision optimally is the question of handling suggestions from your supervisor that require behavioral changes that do not correspond to your natural style. Many students find themselves blocked in this area. They are willing to try to implement suggestions that fit fairly naturally into their style. However, trying something entirely new and out of character is quite a different matter. The issues of fear of evaluation and concern about providing adequate service to the client often keep students comfortably practicing what they already know. You will never broaden yourself as a therapist if you refuse to take risks and try things with which you're uncomfortable. Although you may feel awkward or silly at first, the ability to try new things and the willingness to expose your deficits is crucial to becoming a broadly skilled psychotherapist.

Additional methods of skill attainment

A variety of resources in addition to direct one-to-one supervision are available to the student in training. Students often comment that they find that watching other people do therapy is particularly valuable. This is an interesting yet nonthreatening way of modeling new therapy techniques and interpersonal skills that you may never discover through your own client supervision. We urge students to take advantage of every possible opportunity to watch someone else in action.

We encourage students to watch each other as well as to observe experienced clinicians. However, this appears to be particularly difficult for beginning therapists. This is due partially to the slowness of the therapeutic hour, which is distracting when you're not involved. But more importantly there is a tremendous resistance to watching and commenting on fellow students' work. Students seem to find it threatening to take criticism from one another, and equally difficult to give it. This unfortunate situation is probably a result of the competitive and evaluative atmosphere in which training usually occurs. Students are willing to be supportive to one another but reluctant to accept the evaluator role.

We say this is unfortunate because there is so much to be learned by watching one another and providing feedback and constructive suggestions. You can maximize your own learning by seeking out help from your fellow trainees, even though there is some risk involved. The best way to approach another student is to present him or her with a specific problem or a request for feedback about a difficult situation. You may ask, for example, "I'm having trouble with this. What would you do?" As we've mentioned previously, an outsider with some objectivity and some diversity in skills will often be able to make very useful suggestions. Feeling comfortable about consulting with colleagues will be equally valuable to you after you have completed your training.

Clinical settings usually offer a variety of training opportunities in addition to live or tape modeling of actual therapy sessions. Numerous conferences and workshops are offered by different therapeutic schools and institutes as well as by the professional organizations on both a state and national level. As the movement toward increased continuing education gains momentum in the mental health professions, more and more of these training opportunities will become available to both students and experienced professionals.

Reading books about psychotherapy techniques can be extremely useful in broadening your knowledge and specific skills, even though their actual application in the therapy session will probably need to be discussed with a supervisor experienced in the particular technique. Reading research and case reports in the journal literature may also be helpful. Students often concentrate so hard on learning basic interviewing and therapy skills that they neglect the wealth of information contained in the literature about the techniques and problems they are dealing with. Although this book does not focus on this type of learning, it is essential to make yourself aware of such resources.

The value of personal therapy. Final mention should be made of a matter of some controversy in therapy training, that of personal psychotherapy for the student. Advocates declare that it is essential to have the self-awareness and the perspective on the client role that is afforded by personal experience in therapy. It is claimed that this offers the therapist the most effective opportunity to see another therapist in action. On the other hand, many authorities strongly maintain that it is no more important than any of the other varieties of experience the therapist may or may not share with the client.

We view personal psychotherapy as another educational tool that increases the student's self-awareness and general experience. Although it may not be as essential as closely supervised experience, it can be extremely helpful and even necessary in certain instances to help beginners resolve the problems they encounter in learning to be psychotherapists.

In summary, there are a large variety of ways in which students may improve on their therapy skills, limited almost by the ingenuity of the students themselves. The more and varied your learning efforts are and the more flexibly and openly you approach them, the more you are likely to develop as a mature clinician.

Continued growth

We have written this book for people taking the first steps to becoming therapists and have aimed at presenting some of the needed elementary skills. The therapeutic encounter is a complex situation. Successful therapists must learn to understand and conceptualize a client's problems, to plan treatment strategies, and to communicate effectively. The desire to help people is not sufficient for the student to become an effective clinician. Although our emphasis has been on the initial learning experience, proficiency as a psychotherapist requires continued efforts at skill development throughout your professional career.

Therapeutic abilities improve gradually and unevenly with training and experience. Some skills will change rapidly, whereas others remain stubbornly resistant to alteration. You will probably become deeply discouraged with your inability to conquer a problem, and you may spend several sessions struggling repeatedly with a stylistic deficiency. This is to be expected. You will probably experience great leaps forward and seemingly endless plateaus. You can only be expected to assimilate and implement small amounts of feedback at a time, and students' rates of progress vary tremendously both within and between individuals.

Formal training is only the first step in your professional development as a psychotherapist. Once this phase is complete you face a greater challenge. You are no longer formally evaluated or observed in your work. It is easy to become isolated and somewhat rigid and stagnant in your approach. It takes commitment to continue growth, to work at acquiring new knowledge, and to remain open to new ideas. There are many avenues available for pursuing this goal. In truth your education as a therapist should never be considered complete. Throughout your professional career you will find yourself changing, learning, and adding to your array of therapeutic skills.

211

Suggested reading

We have listed a number of resources that students have found helpful in supplementing clinical supervision during their practicum training. The list is not intended to be comprehensive or exhaustive. Useful resources available to students far outnumber this brief listing. However, we have specified certain books that either supply information in greater depth or represent a different point of view from that presented in this book.

Annon, Jack. *The behavioral treatment of sexual problems.* Vols. I & II. Honolulu: Enabling Systems, 1974 & 1975. A comprehensive review of sex therapy with many excellent clinical examples.

Balsam, R. M., & Balsam, A. *Becoming a psychotherapist: a clinical primer.* Boston: Little, Brown, and Company, 1974. Balsam and Balsam address the problems and issues that arise during psychoanalytic psychotherapy training but that have some broader applicability to students training in other fields. The clinical examples described are particularly interesting.

Bellak, L., & Small, L. *Emergency psychotherapy and brief psychotherapy.* New York: Grune & Stratton, Inc., 1965. A more in-depth coverage of crisis intervention techniques than we were able to provide in one chapter. Also covers the considerations important in short-term psychotherapy.

Benjamin, A. *The helping interview.* (2nd ed.) Boston: Houghton Mifflin Company, 1974. This is an in-depth examination of the interviewing process from a nondirective, humanistic view. It is valuable in providing specific suggestions about how to gather information and how to communicate effectively and empathetically with a client.

Bergen, A. E. & Strupp, H. H. *Changing frontiers in the science of psychotherapy.* Chicago: Aldine Publishing Company, 1972. A collection of research articles that focus on a variety of specific treatment approaches and evaluate their effectiveness. Gives a broad overview of different approaches. Points out some of the issues discussed in the chapter on skill attainment.

Bockar, Joyce A. *Primer for the nonmedical therapist.* Holliswood, N.Y.: Spectrum Publications, Inc., 1976. This is a very useful book that acquaints nonmedical psychotherapists with a basic knowledge of (1) illnesses with psychophysiological components and (2) specific knowledge of drugs most commonly used by psychotherapy clients.

Ellis, Albert. *Growth through reason.* Palo Alto, Calif.: Science & Behavior Books, 1971. Theoretical presentation and verbatim transcripts of rational emotive therapy sessions with clients.

Ellis, Albert. *Humanistic psychotherapy: the rational emotive approach.* New York: Julian Press, Inc., 1973. This book provides a good summary of the theoretical development of rational-emotive therapy as well as its application to clinical problems.

Gilmore, S. K. *The counselor-in-training.* New York: Prentice-Hall, Inc., 1973. This is an excellent practicum training text but is limited in its applicability to counseling (rather than clinical) settings and purposes. It provides both a broad conceptual framework for understanding the task of counseling and structured exercises for classroom training.

Goldfried, Marvin R., & Davison, Gerald C. *Clinical behavior therapy.* New York: Holt, Rinehart and Winston, Inc., 1976. Descriptions of behavioral techniques and how they are applied to clinical problems.

Gottman, J. M. and Leiblum, S. R. *How to do psychotherapy and how to evaluate it.* New York: Holt, Rinehart and Winston, Inc., 1974. This book is written from a cognitive-behavioral point of view and is of use almost exclusively for behavioral treatment. It is practical and emphasizes a conceptual framework for evaluation of effectiveness of treatment.

Greenson, Ralph. *The technique and practice of psychoanalysis.* New York: International Universities Press, 1967. Description of commonly encountered clinical problems and examples of ways a psychoanalytic clinician would respond to them.

Kaplan, H. S. *The new sex therapy.* New York: Brunner/Mazel, Inc., 1974. Specific techniques useful in the practice of sexual treatment. Problem oriented and specific, this text provides extensive theoretical material on the development and maintenance of sexual problems.

Lazarus, Arnold A. *Behavior therapy and beyond.* New York: McGraw-Hill Book Company, 1971. One of the first books to address the practical concerns of learning to do therapy, it takes a cognitive-behavioral point of view and has extensive examples from the author's experience with clients.

Lederer, W. J., & Jackson, D. D. *The mirages of marriage.* New York: W. W. Norton & Company, Inc., 1968. This book is a good resource for therapists working with couples experiencing marital problems. It is theoretically based on the "systems" concept, which focuses on the impact of the interacting communications network operating in the family unit.

Leitenberg, Harold. *Handbook of behavior modification and behavior therapy.* Englewood Cliffs, N.J.: Prentice-Hall, Inc., 1976. Review of theoretical and empirical studies of behavior approaches to a number of applied areas.

London, Perry. *The modes and morals of psychotherapy.* New York: Holt, Rinehart and Winston, Inc., 1964. Good, helpful, and stimulating discussion of ethical and professional considerations that are only highlighted in our book.

Menninger, Karl. *Theory of psychoanalytic technique.* New York: Harper & Row, Publishers, 1958. Classic work on the principles of the psychoanalytic approach.

Patterson, Gerald. *Families.* Champaign, Ill.: Research Press, 1971. A behavioral approach to family therapy.

Rogers, Carl R. *Client centered therapy.* Boston: Houghton Mifflin Company, 1951. This classic work outlines the basic theoretical underpinnings and clinical principles of the client-centered school of psychotherapy.

Satir, V. *Conjoint family therapy.* (Rev. ed.) Palo Alto, Calif.: Science and Behavior Books, 1967. Satir offers a very popular conceptual view of the problems of children and families, including many specific treatment suggestions in an informal training manual format.

Shelton, John L., & Ackerman, J. Mark. *Homework in counseling and psychotherapy.* Springfield, Ill.: Charles C Thomas, Publisher, 1974. Practical, technique-oriented book promoting the idea that therapy can have broader effects if used in conjunction with systematic homework assignments. Most applicable to behavioral and cognitive therapies.

Simmon, James E. *Psychiatric examination of children.* Philadelphia: Lea & Febiger, 1974. Some hints for interviewing children and adolescents.

Sullivan, H. S. *The psychiatric interview.* New York: W. W. Norton & Company, Inc., 1970. Sullivan's lectures are a sophisticated, psychodynamically oriented discussion of the interview. The book is complex and often brilliant but not recommended as a text for beginners.

Weiner, Irving B. *Principles of psychotherapy.* New York: John Wiley & Sons, Inc., 1975. This is a detailed manual describing the psychotherapy process, primarily from a psychodynamic point of view, that relates available research findings to clinical applications.

Woodruff, R. A., Goodwin, D. W., & Guze, S. B. *Psychiatric diagnosis.* New York: Oxford University Press, 1974. This is a useful reference for students who are expected to use the psychiatric system of classification in their clinical work. It provides helpful information about classification in general and about the specific diagnoses referenced in the *Diagnostic and Statistical Manual II.*

Yalom, Irvin D. *Theory and practice of group psychotherapy.* New York: Basic Books, Inc., 1970. This is a comprehensive handbook that gives a broad overview of group therapy and guidance for the training of group therapists.